DIAGNOSTIC PICTURE TESTS IN

ORAL MEDICINE

W.R. Tyldesley
DDS, PhD, MSc, FDSRCS

Director of Dental Education
University of Liverpool, England

Wolfe Medical Publications Ltd

Titles in this series, published or being developed, include:

Diagnostic Picture Tests in Paediatrics

Picture Tests in Human Anatomy

Diagnostic Picture Tests in Oral Medicine

Diagnostic Picture Tests in Orthopaedics

Diagnostic Picture Tests in Infectious Diseases

Diagnostic Picture Tests in Dermatology

Diagnostic Picture Tests in Ophthalmology

Diagnostic Picture Tests in Rheumatology

Diagnostic Picture Tests in Obstetrics/Gynaecology

Diagnostic Picture Tests in Neurology

Diagnostic Picture Tests in Sports Injuries

Picture Tests in Surgical Diagnosis

Copyright © W.R. Tyldesley, 1986
Published by Wolfe Medical Publications Ltd, 1986
Printed by BPCC Hazell Books, Aylesbury, England
ISBN 0 7234 0937 4
Reprinted 1988, 1991

For full details of all Wolfe titles please write to
Wolfe Publishing Ltd, Brook House, 2–16 Torrington Place,
London WC1E 7LT, England.

Coventry University

Preface

The patients presented in this collection are representative of those seen in the Oral Medicine clinic and (naturally) predominantly demonstrate lesions of the oral mucosa. However, in such a clinic a wide range of patients is seen and so a number of conditions are included which might be reasonably classified under the heading of 'Oral Surgery' if a pedantic attitude were adopted. Oral medicine is a discipline which is essentially diagnostic and depends to a great extent upon the various investigative procedures following initial clinical examination. None the less, the initial provisional clinical diagnosis based upon observation and careful history-taking remains the most important single factor in the investigation of a patient.

The questions (and answers) reflect this view – most of the answers are arranged to emphasise the significance of full investigation on the future management of the patient. It is strongly recommended that the reader's own answers should be written down in brief note form before the answers given in the text are consulted – it is all too easy to assume, after turning to the printed answer, a more complete response in oneself than in fact occurred. The cases are presented in completely random order with no attempt at gradation.

The majority of the patients illustrated have been referred to and seen by the author in his clinics. Professor John Lemmer and Dr T.W. Stewart have kindly allowed the use of illustrations of their patients.

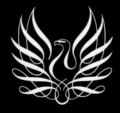

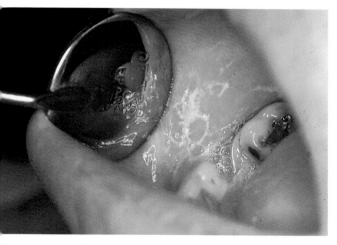

1 A typical oral lesion seen in a disease of the skin.
(a) What is the disease?
(b) What other types of oral lesions may appear?
(c) What treatment is available for this type of lesion?
(d) What is its association with generalised disease processes?
(e) Has it potential for malignant transformation?

2 The appearance of the anterior teeth in a relatively young female patient.
(a) What is the abnormality?
(b) What mechanism may lead to this abnormality?
(c) Which generalised conditions may be associated?

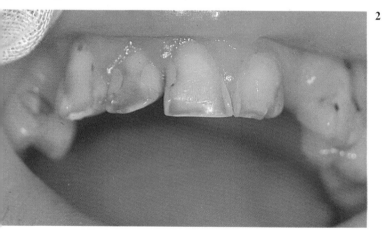

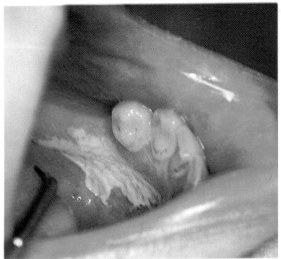

3 A symptom free lesion of the floor of the mouth.
(a) What is the clinical diagnosis?
(b) What action should be taken?
(c) What is the prognosis of such a lesion?

4 This firm, pain free, slowly growing swelling is in the palate of a middle aged patient. There are no radiographic changes.
(a) What might this lesion be?
(b) What action should be taken?

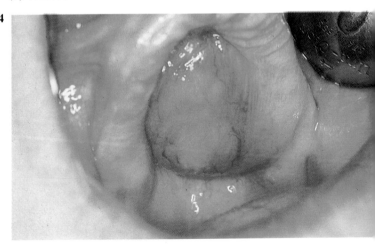

5, 6 The lesion of the chin (**5**) appeared in the patient whose dental condition is shown in **6**.
(a) What might the skin lesion be?
(b) What further investigation should be conducted?
(c) What definitive action should be taken?

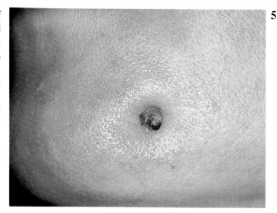

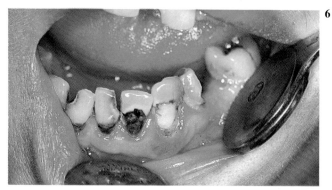

7 A painless defect of the palate of some years' standing in a 90-year-old patient.
(a) What is the most likely diagnosis?
(b) What diagnostic procedures should be carried out?
(c) Is treatment indicated?

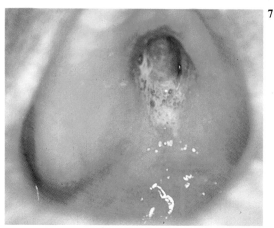

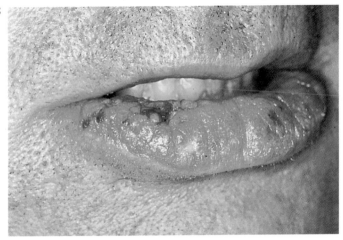

8 A middle-aged male has worked as a farmer in Australia for most of his life.
(a) What might be the diagnosis of the lower lip lesion?
(b) How is the personal history of this patient significant?
(c) Is it a significant lesion?

9 These teeth show hypoplastic features.
(a) At what stage of development did the abnormality occur?
(b) What may cause the hypoplasia?
(c) Are such teeth unusually susceptible to caries?
(d) Does this condition affect both permanent and deciduous teeth?

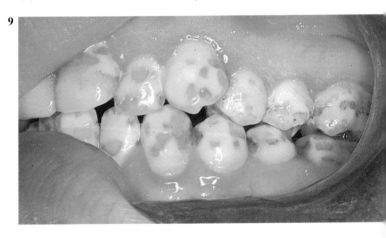

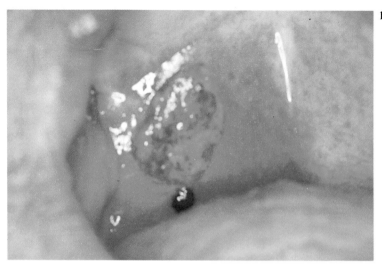

10 A patient complained of 'blood blisters' on the palate.
(a) What diagnoses should be initially considered?
(b) Which special investigations should be conducted?
(c) How can blister formation be prevented?

11 A painless, slow-growing, unilateral bony swelling of the maxilla in a 12-year-old patient.
(a) What is the most likely diagnosis?
(b) What are the probable results of a biochemical blood screen?
(c) What treatment is indicated?

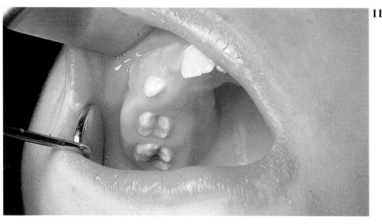

12

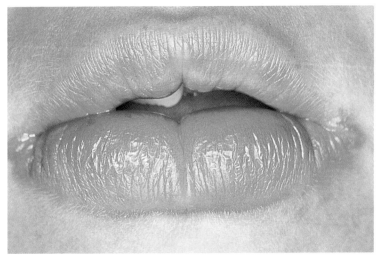

12 A ten-year-old patient developed swelling of the lower lip with angular cheilitis.
(a) Which gastrointestinal tract disease could this indicate?
(b) What other oral lesions may be present?
(c) What investigations are needed to confirm the diagnosis?
(d) Might the oral condition present without findings in the gastrointestinal tract?

13

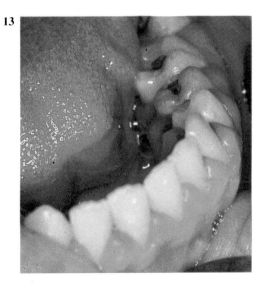

13 A 22-year-old female complained of recent enlargement of the gingivae with a minor degree of bleeding and feeling generally unwell.
(a) What is the most important differential diagnosis?
(b) What immediate steps should be taken?
(c) What other possible diagnosis at once comes to mind?

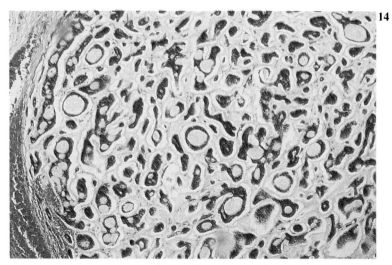

14 Histological appearance of a painless slow-growing lump in the palate.
(a) What is the diagnosis?
(b) What is the clinical significance?
(c) What further steps should follow biopsy?

15 An Indian lady complained of increasing difficulty in opening her mouth. A previous period of oral ulceration is now in remission. The irregularity on the buccal mucosa has a firm fibrous texture.
(a) What is the most likely diagnosis?
(b) What is the aetiology?
(c) How is it treated?

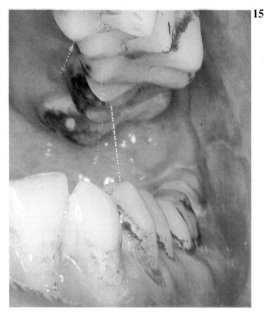

16 Oral lesions appeared suddenly after a few days of medical treatment for a middle-aged lady's rheumatoid arthritis.
(a) What may have caused the lesions?
(b) What diagnostic step is particularly helpful?
(c) What is the treatment?

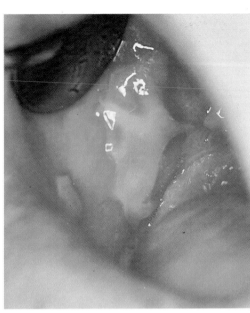

17 An elderly male underwent a subtotal gastrectomy some years ago.
(a) What might be the connection between this lesion and the gastrectomy?
(b) What investigations are necessary?
(c) What treatment should be carried out?

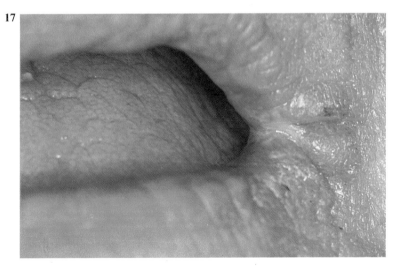

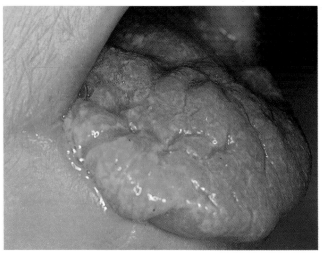

18 The patient suffers from myasthenia gravis.
(a) What is the oral lesion?
(b) What other associated abnormality may be present?
(c) What is the treatment for the oral lesion?

19 A salivary gland demonstrated by contrast radiography.
(a) Which gland is involved?
(b) What is the most obvious feature?
(c) What might be the cause?

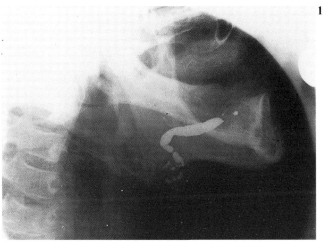

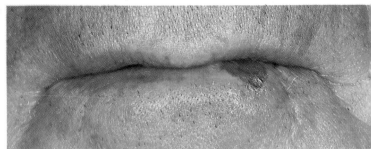

20 A 60-year-old man complained of a non-healing 'cold sore' on his lower lip.
(a) What important diagnosis should be considered?
(b) Why are his personal details important?
(c) What is the approach to therapy?

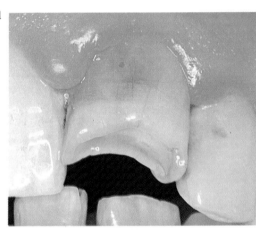

21 (a) What is the characteristic appearance of the left upper central incisor?
(b) What is the aetiology?
(c) What clinical evidence confirms the aetiology?

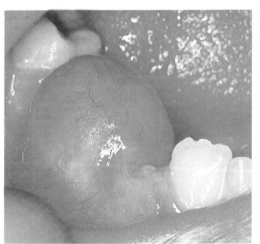

22 A painless swelling occurred suddenly in an 11-year-old girl.
(a) What might it be?
(b) What steps should be taken?
(c) What is the structure of the cyst wall?

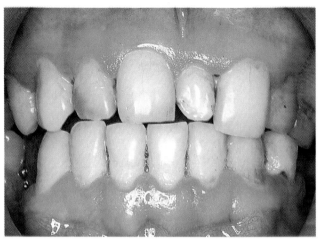

23 (a) What is illustrated in this adult male?
(b) Is the condition associated with other dental anomalies?
(c) Is it more common in primary or secondary dentition?

24 (a) What is the lesion in this middle-aged male?
(b) What is the clinical significance of this kind of lesion?
(c) What steps should be taken?

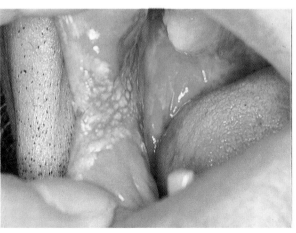

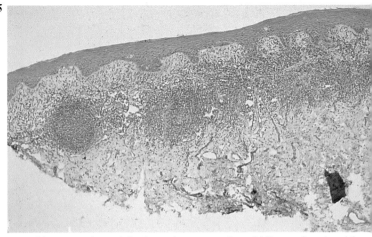

25 A biopsy section of the buccal mucosa of a middle-aged male with suspected lichen planus.
(a) What is the unusual appearance?
(b) How is it significant?
(c) What further investigations are called for?

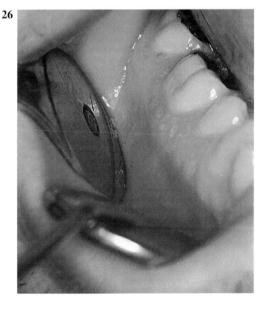

26 A 30-year-old male complained of recurrent, moderately uncomfortable, small blisters of the oral mucosa, particularly affecting the gingivae, Herpes simplex virus particles were positively identified in samples taken from the lesions.
(a) What might be this condition?
(b) Is this a common situation?
(c) What further investigations should be conducted?

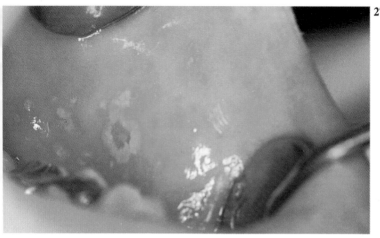

27, 28 These lesions appeared in a young male complaining only of mild discomfort and slight malaise.
(a) What might be this condition?
(b) What infective agent may be involved?
(c) How might the diagnosis be confirmed?
(d) What action should be taken?

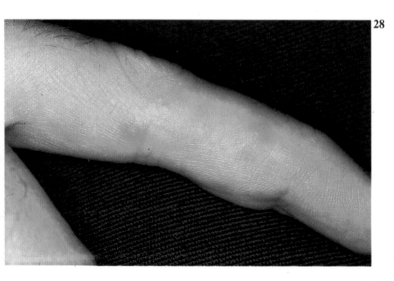

29

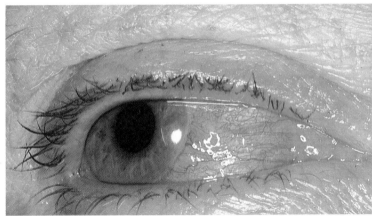

29 This man had suffered from oral and genital ulceration for some years.
(a) What might be the eye lesion?
(b) What steps should be taken?
(c) What HLA markers may be associated?

30 The patient complained of intermittent soreness of the tongue.
(a) What is the condition?
(b) What is its aetiology?
(c) What investigations should be carried out?
(d) How is it treated?

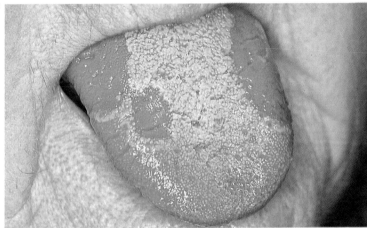

31 (a) What is the condition in this middle-aged edentulous woman?
(b) What aetiological factors should be considered?
(c) What organisms are likely to be involved?
(d) What other lesion is likely to be associated?

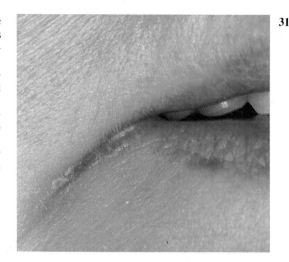

31

32, 33 The lesion (**32**) was present in a 25-year-old female. There were minimal bone changes on X-ray. The histology is seen in **33**.
(a) What is the lesion?
(b) With what generalised disease process might it be associated?
(c) What further investigations are advisable?
(d) What abnormal results might be significant?
(e) What neoplasm might be present in another site?

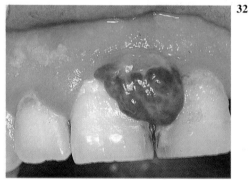

32

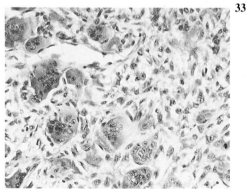

33

34

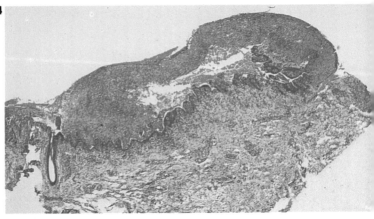

34 This section (stained H&E) is from a blistering lesion in the palate in a 50-year-old Jewish patient.
(a) What kind of lesion is it?
(b) What is the clinical diagnosis?
(c) To confirm the diagnosis what histological technique could be employed?
(d) Why is this an important diagnosis?
(e) What is the significance of the personal details?

35 An extremely painful lesion on a dentist's finger.
(a) What is its relationship with the lesion in **36**?
(b) What steps should be taken?

35

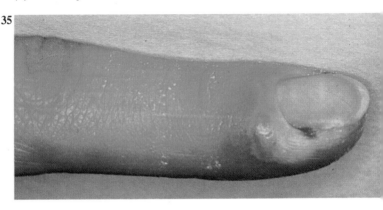

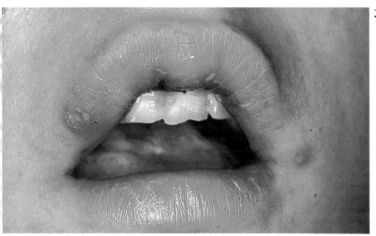

36 A 19-year-old female had complained of malaise and submandibular tenderness over two days.
(a) What is the likely diagnosis?
(b) What key factor in the clinical history would confirm this possibility?
(c) What laboratory investigations would help in the confirmation?
(d) What is the eventual outcome?

37 The badly affected eye of a patient with bullous lesions in the mouth.
(a) What might be this condition?
(b) In what order do the lesions present?
(c) What is the technique used to define the diagnosis?
(d) What might be expected as the result of such an investigation?

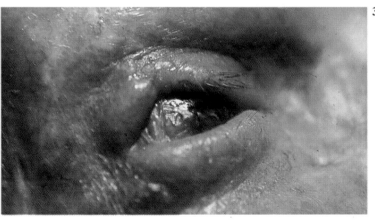

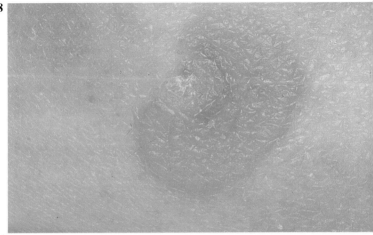

38 A lesion appeared on the forearm of a 20-year-old patient with a history of recurrent stomatitis.
(a) What might be the lesion?
(b) What diagnosis does it imply?
(c) What precipitating factors may be present?

39

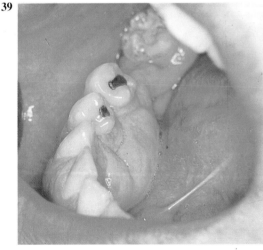

39 The symptom-free gingival enlargement has been present for as long as the patient can remember. It has a fibrous consistency. There are similar changes in other quadrants.
(a) What might it be?
(b) Is it associated with any other abnormality?
(c) What systemic investigations should be made?
(d) What is the approach to treatment?

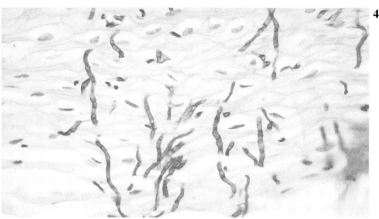

40 Section (stained PAS) from a biopsy of a leukoplakia on the buccal mucosa.
(a) What is the most evident feature?
(b) How is this significant?
(c) How might it affect management of the lesion?

41 The lesion appeared relatively quickly in an elderly female.
(a) What might it be?
(b) What other oral lesions might be present which would help to confirm the clinical diagnosis?
(c) What further diagnostic steps should be taken?
(d) What is the significance of the personal details?

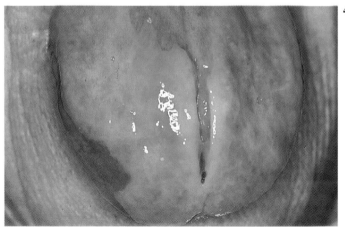

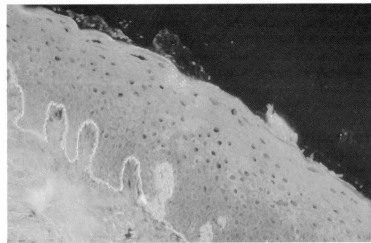

42 A section from tissue adjacent to a blistering lesion of the palate, stained by immunofluorescent techniques to demonstrate the presence of antibody complexes (IgG class).
(a) What type of lesion is likely to form?
(b) What might be the diagnosis?

43 A middle-aged female with severe rheumatoid arthritis developed an anterior open bite over a period of less than a year.
(a) What is the cause?
(b) What is the prognosis?
(c) What action should be taken?

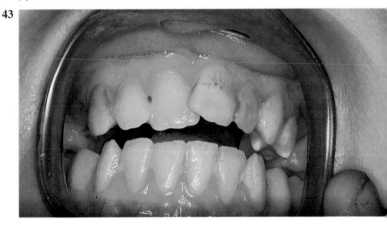

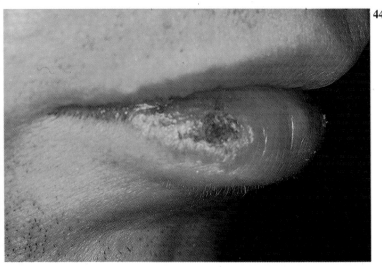

44, 45 The lesion (**44**) appeared on the lip of a patient with a light-sensitive rash over the bridge of the nose (**45**).
(a) What might be the condition?
(b) With what might the lesion be clinically confused?
(c) What histology would be shown on biopsy of the lip?
(d) What is the prognosis?

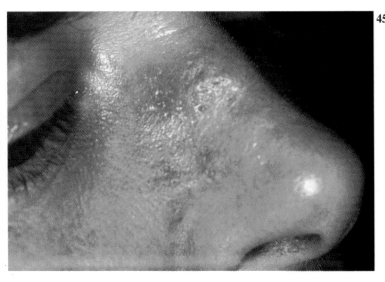

46

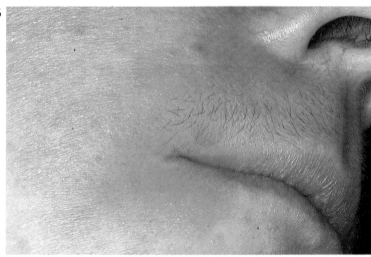

46 (a) What might be the rash in this 20-year-old female?
(b) Why are the personal details significant?
(c) What is the aetiology?
(d) Should it be treated by steroids?

47 A painful ulcer appeared quite rapidly in a 12-year-old girl.
(a) What might this be?
(b) What action should be taken?

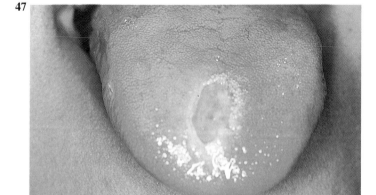

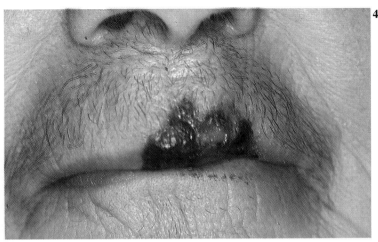

48 A lip lesion appeared on a middle-aged female taking high doses of systemic steroids.
(a) What might it be?
(b) What organisms might be involved?
(c) What investigations should be conducted?
(d) What action is necessary?

49 A 20-year-old female felt ill for a few days. She had swollen cervical nodes and an elevated temperature.
(a) What is the most likely diagnosis?
(b) What important differential diagnosis must be considered?
(c) What initial diagnostic step is therefore essential?
(d) What misleading finding might be present in the result of the test?

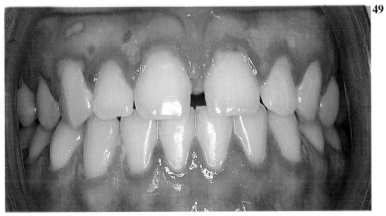

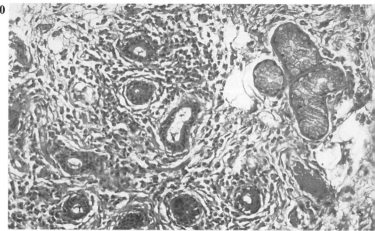

50 A section from a labial gland biopsy of a 60-year-old female complaining of a dry mouth.
(a) What are the significant appearances?
(b) What other examinations should be carried out?
(c) What is the prognosis of the dry mouth?

51 (a) In this poorly controlled diabetic patient, what might be the mucosal lesion?
(b) What other oral abnormalities may occur?
(c) What may be the effect on the salivary glands?

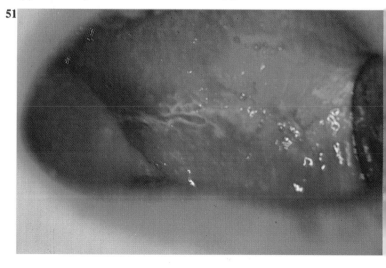

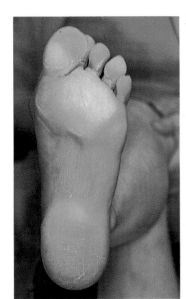

52, 53 (a) What is the condition in **52** of this 40-year-old female?
(b) What is the connection with the oral lesion in **53**?
(c) What other condition may be involved?
(d) What genetic factors are involved?
(e) What other oral abnormality may be associated?

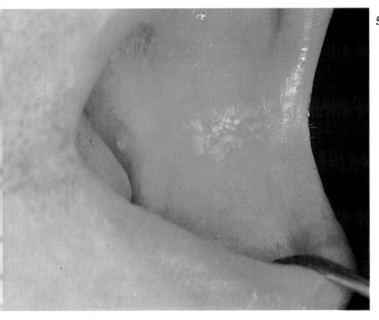

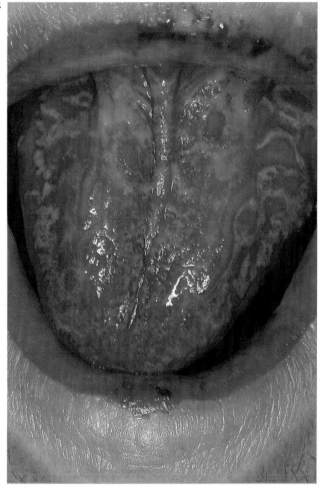

54 The patient has been treated for ulceration of the tongue.
(a) What is to be seen?
(b) Is this the result of reasonable treatment?
(c) Are there any dangers implicit in this treatment?

55 (a) What abnormality is illustrated in this 50-year-old lady with rheumatoid arthritis?
(b) What other complaints might be associated?
(c) What is the syndrome involved?
(d) What other process might have resulted in the same condition?

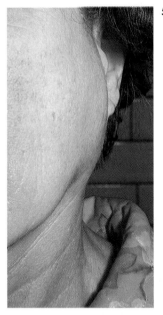

56 (a) What is the obvious abnormality in the anterior teeth of this ten-year-old girl?
(b) At what stage of development did this occur?
(c) Is there any obvious cause?

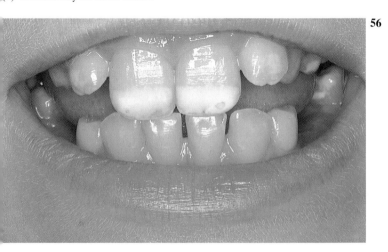

57

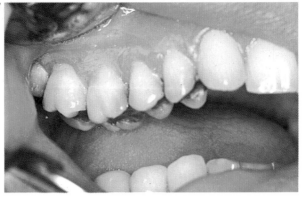

57, 58 The gingival lesions are in 35-year-old females.
(a) What is the relationship between the lesions?
(b) What is the significance of the personal details?
(c) How can the clinical diagnosis be confirmed?
(d) What alternative clinical diagnosis should be considered in **58**?
(e) What clinical term describes the condition in **58**?

58

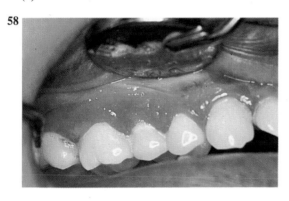

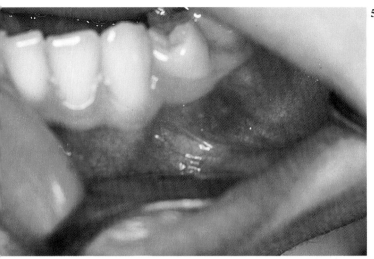

59 This symptom-free lesion was found on routine examination.
(a) What diagnoses come to mind?
(b) What investigations should be carried out?
(c) What action should be taken?

60 This condition has recurred on several occasions.
(a) What might it be?
(b) What other structures may be involved?
(c) What group of patients is most likely to be affected?
(d) What is the long term prognosis?
(e) What type of therapy is used?

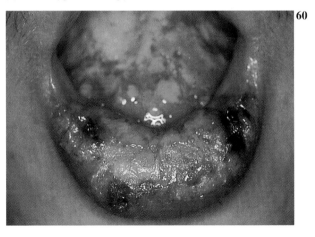

61

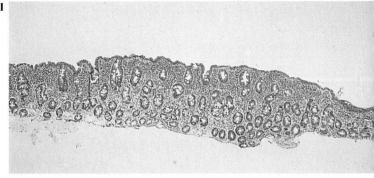

62

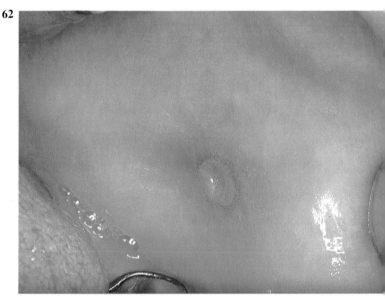

61, 62 A section (**61**) from a jejunal biopsy of the patient with recurrent oral ulceration in **62**.

(a) What is the abnormality in the section?
(b) What is the relationship between this and the oral ulceration?
(c) What special characteristics are shown by the oral ulceration?
(d) What is the cause of the jejunal abnormality?
(e) What steps should be taken?

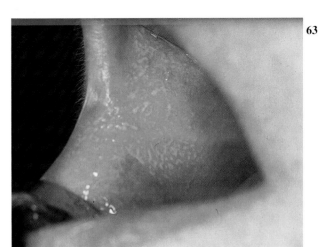

63 A symptom free condition in a middle-aged female.
(a) What might it be?
(b) With what may it be confused on superficial clinical examination?
(c) What action is necessary?

64 (a) What is this slightly irritable lesion of the tongue?
(b) What action should be taken?

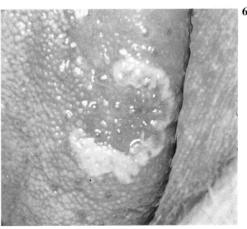

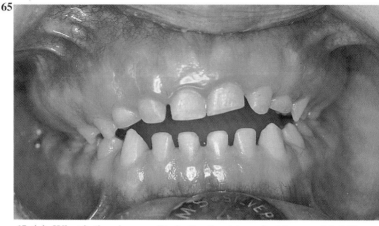

65 (a) What is the abnormality in the dentition of a 16-year-old girl?
(b) With what might it be confused initially?
(c) What generalised factors may be associated?

66 A 17-year-old girl has systemic lupus erythematosus.
(a) What might be the oral lesions?
(b) What treatment should be adopted?

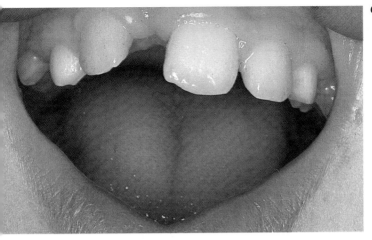

67 (a) What is the obvious abnormality in this eight-year-old child?
(b) What is its most common cause?
(c) What steps should be taken?

68 This patient has oral lichen planus.
(a) What might be the white lip lesion?
(b) What action should be taken?
(c) What other lip lesions may occur?

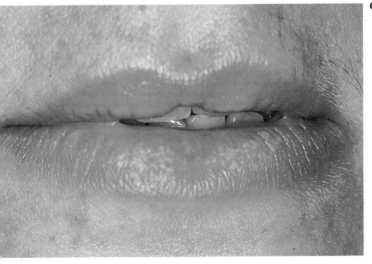

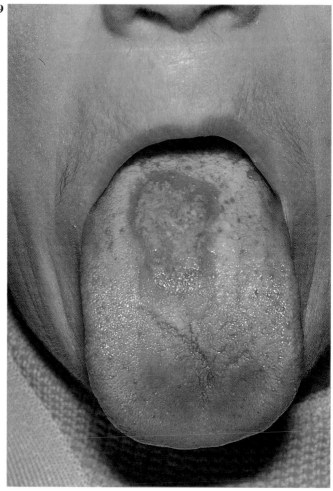

69 The lesion of the tongue is painless.
(a) What might it be?
(b) What is the important infective factor?
(c) What treatment is indicated?

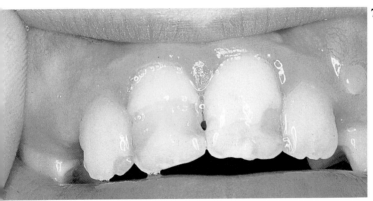

70 The teeth of a 13-year-old boy with recurrent oral ulceration. His father has a flat jejunal mucosa, found during investigation for recurrent oral ulceration.
(a) What abnormality is present?
(b) When during development did this abnormality occur?
(c) What is its significance in the present circumstances?
(d) What further investigations should be carried out?

71 An 11-year-old girl felt ill for two or three days. She had tender palpable cervical nodes.
(a) What is the most significant possible diagnosis?
(b) What is the most likely differential diagnosis?
(c) What investigation should be carried out immediately?
(d) What error may be involved in the interpretation?

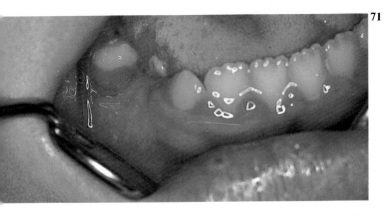

72

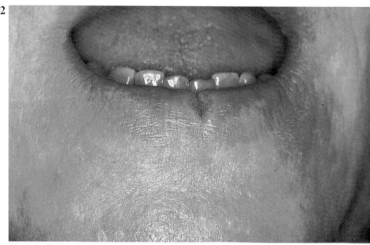

72 (a) What is the lesion on the lower lip of this 30-year-old male?
(b) What infective element may be present?
(c) How should this be treated?

73 A painful lesion in a 65-year-old male.
(a) What might it be?
(b) What action should be taken?
(c) What is the significance of the personal details?

73

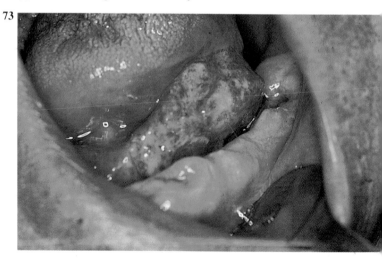

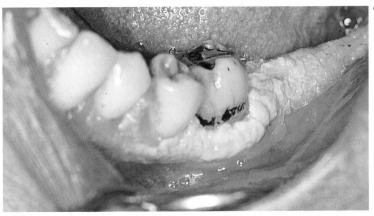

74 A lesion found on routine dental examination.
(a) What is it?
(b) What might be the aetiology?
(c) What steps should be taken?

75 A young female has persistent, painful, recurrent oral ulceration, predominantly affecting the margins and underside of the tongue.
(a) What variant of recurrent oral ulceration is this?
(b) What are its most characteristic features?
(c) What is its response to treatment?
(d) What investigations should be carried out?

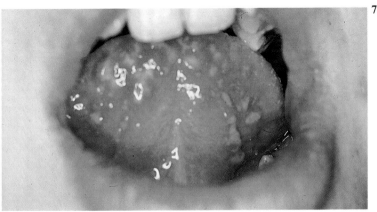

76

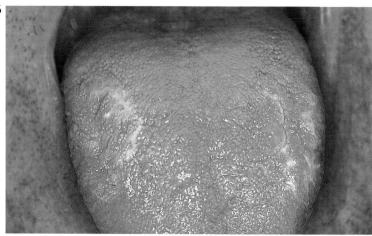

76 (a) What might be the lesions in this 50-year-old male?
(b) What is an alternative clinical diagnosis?
(c) What other lesions may be present?

77 A typical field from the blood film of a young patient complaining of a sore mouth and bleeding from the gingivae.
(a) What is the probable diagnosis?
(b) What oral lesions may be involved at an early stage?
(c) What is the reason for the gingival bleeding?

77

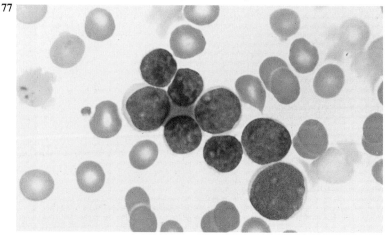

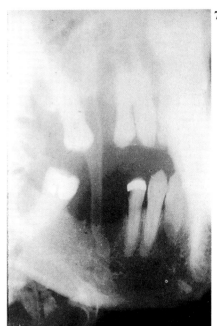

78

78, 79 The radiograph demonstrates an uncommon, but quite well known, cause of oro-facial pain.
(a) What is the bony abnormality?
(b) What is the soft tissue lesion in **79** which may result from this?
(c) What is the distribution of pain?
(d) What is the approach to treatment?

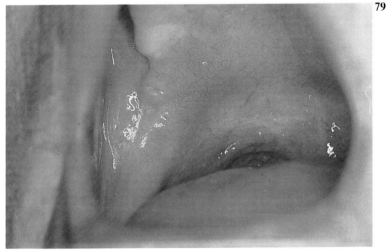

79

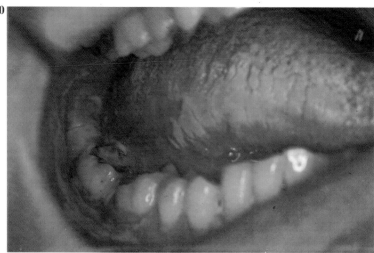

80 After suffering from severe toothache for several days, this patient had attempted to self-treat.
(a) What might be the abnormality of the mucosa?
(b) What is the relationship between this mucosal lesion and the nearby teeth?
(c) What should be done about it?

81 (a) What might be this lesion in the palate of a 55-year-old male?
(b) What aetiological factors might be involved?
(c) What is the prognosis?

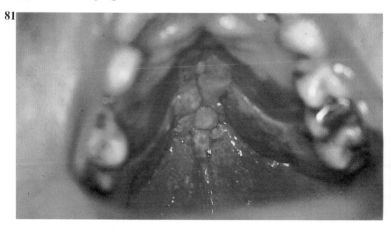

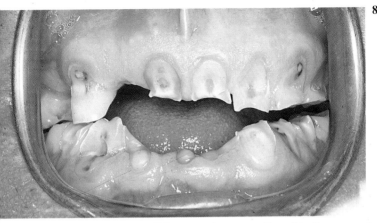

82 (a) What three classic conditions may have contributed to the unusual dental state of this 50-year-old man?
(b) What generalised disturbance may be involved in such an advanced case of tooth substance loss?

83 A very painful lesion on the tongue of a patient with ulcerative colitis.
(a) What might it be?
(b) What similar lesion may appear on the skin?
(c) What are their origins?
(d) What other oral lesions may occur which parallel those on the skin?
(e) What other oral lesions may occur in ulcerative colitis?

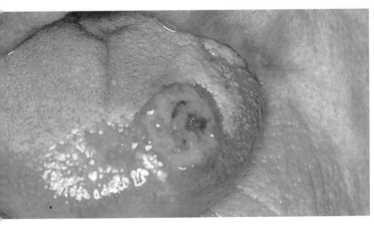

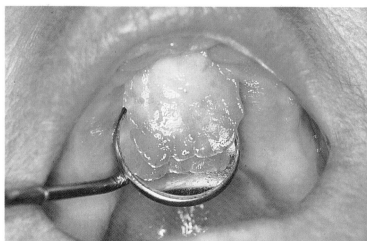

84 A completely asymptomatic lesion found below an upper denture.
(a) What is it and what other names are used?
(b) Why is there this difference in nomenclature?
(c) What is the treatment?

85 A 60-year-old complaining of a sore tongue, angular cheilitis and loss
of energy for some months, had haemoglobin and erythrocyte values
within normal limits.
(a) What other investigations should be carried out?
(b) What abnormalities might be shown?

85

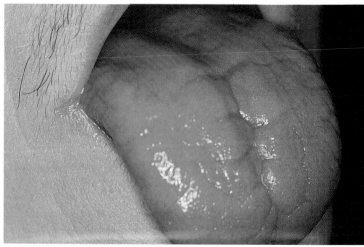

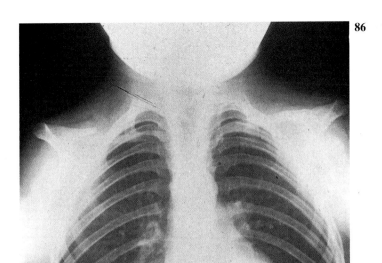

86, 87 Radiographs characteristic of a patient with a well known but uncommon condition.
(a) What might it be?
(b) What are the components of this syndrome?
(c) What are the dental problems?
(d) What is its genetic basis?

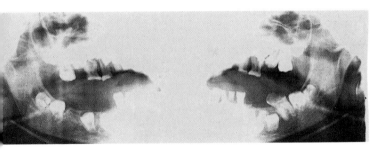

88

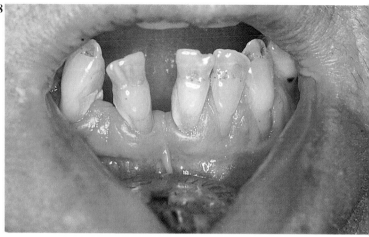

88 The patient had rickets as a child.
(a) What is rickets?
(b) What deficiency is involved?
(c) What is the likelihood of dental abnormalities?
(d) What is the equivalent adult condition?

89 The patient is in the mixed dentition stage.
(a) What is the most obvious abnormality?
(b) Is this more common in the deciduous or the permanent dentition?
(c) Which region of the dentition is most commonly affected?

89

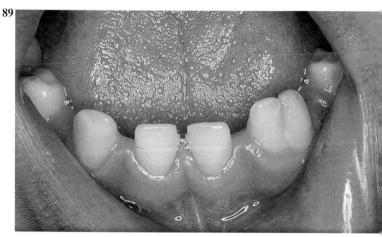

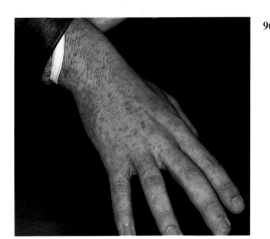

90 This man, with irritable skin lesions, had been prescribed ampicillin for an oral infection.
(a) Should this be thought of as a reaction to penicillins in general?
(b) What condition is said to be particularly involved in this reaction?

91 A blood film from a patient with a sore tongue and angular cheilitis.
(a) What abnormality is shown?
(b) What further tests should be carried out?
(c) What is the most likely diagnosis?

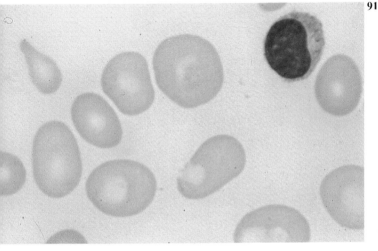

92

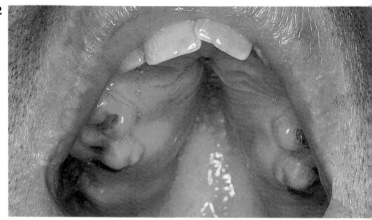

92 The bony enlargement of the alveolar bone of a 30-year-old male is apparently static.
(a) What might this be?
(b) What systemic associations might it have?
(c) What action should be taken?

93 (a) What condition is shown in this adult male?
(b) With what generalised conditions might it be associated?
(c) Is this condition common in the primary dentition?
(d) In cases in which only a few teeth are affected, which are these likely to be?

93

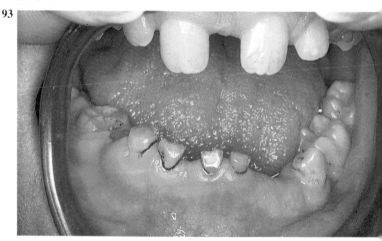

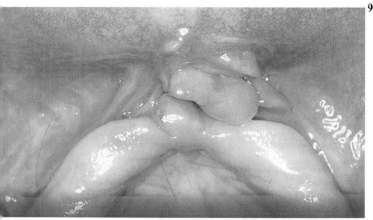

94 The patient has been edentulous for many years.
a) What is the lesion?
b) What is its essential nature?
c) What is its malignant potential?

95 The slow-growing lesion on this tongue is painless.
a) What might it be?
b) Is it in a common site?
c) What is the treatment?

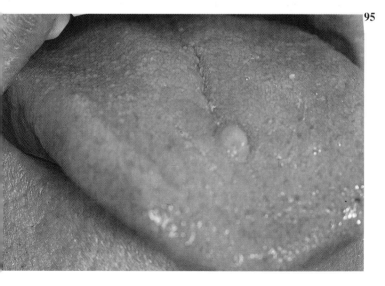

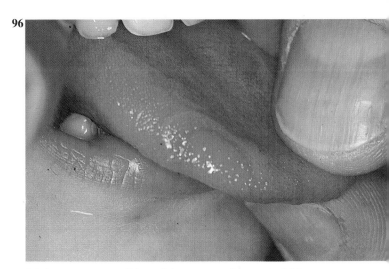

96 A recurrent condition of the tongue of a young child.
(a) What might it be?
(b) Is it rare in this age group?
(c) Is it painful?
(d) What are the systemic implications?

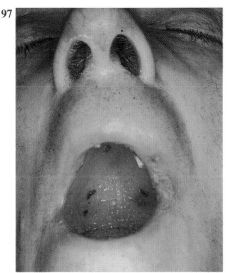

97 A middle-aged male patient felt ill.
(a) What is this?
(b) What might be its cause?
(c) What is the most significant eventual diagnosis?
(d) What other insignificant diagnosis may be involved?

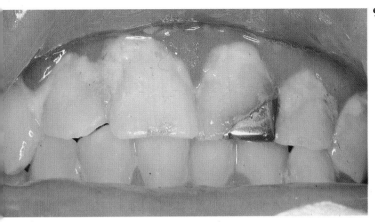

98 (a) What is the condition in this adult male?
(b) What are the clinical signs and symptoms?
(c) What is its cause?
(d) What organisms are involved?
(e) What generalised diseases might be involved?

99 (a) What is this important investigative procedure?
(b) In what conditions of the head and neck might it be valuable?
(c) In what structure is the lesion (marked T)?

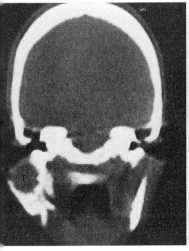
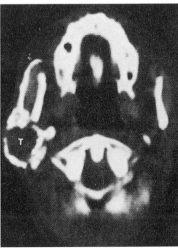

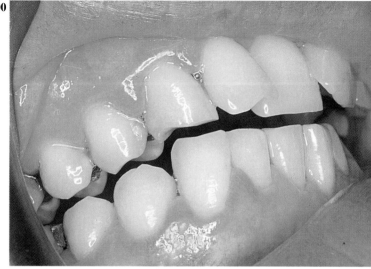

100 In this condition of the teeth on the right side of the mouth there is associated left-sided facial pain, earache and headache.
(a) What is it?
(b) What is the possible association with the facial pain?
(c) Is it a common association?

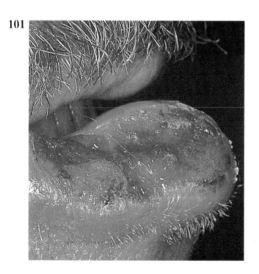

101 (a) What is the most likely diagnosis of this lesion in a 65-year-old man?
(b) What is the prognosis?
(c) What is the ratio between males and females with this condition?
(d) What is the ratio between such lesions on the upper and lower lips?

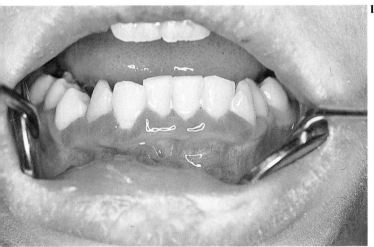

102 A 15-year-old girl had several attacks of painful oral ulceration and gingivitis at approximately monthly intervals when she also had neutropenia.
a) What might this be?
b) What further investigations are required?
c) What is the basic mechanism involved?
d) What is the most common cause of neutropenia in young patients?

103 The lesion on the tongue is painless.
a) What is the clinical diagnosis?
b) What important differential diagnosis must be considered?
c) Should biopsy be performed?
d) What treatment should be considered?

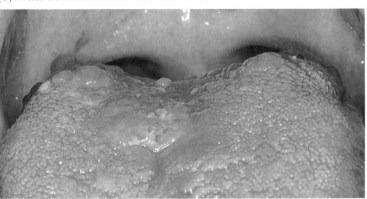

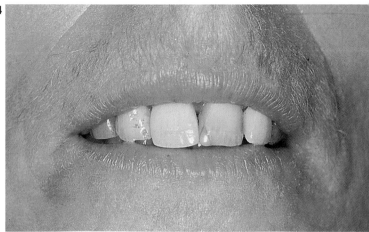

104 (a) What might be the connective tissue disease in this patient?
(b) What other oral changes have been described?
(c) Which is the predominant sex in this disease?

105 (a) What is the obvious abnormality in this 30-year-old patient?
(b) What is its cause?
(c) Is this a common situation?

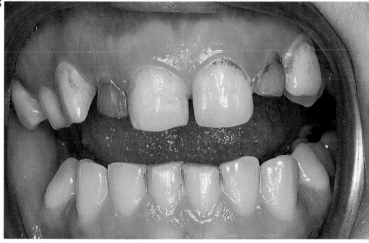

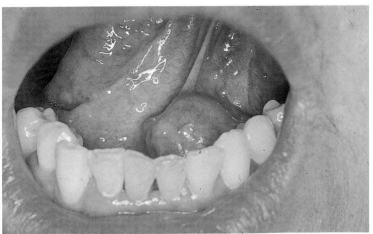

106 An adult patient with intermittent swelling of the floor of the mouth.
(a) What might it be?
(b) What is its most common cause?
(c) What investigations should be conducted?
(d) What is the basis of treatment?

107 (a) What is this lesion in the palate of a middle-aged man?
(b) What is the precise causative factor?
(c) What is the prognosis?
(d) What other lesions should be looked for?

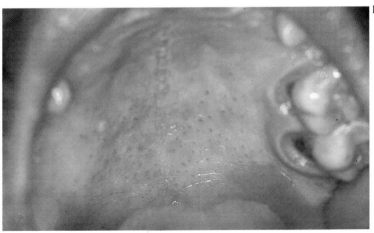

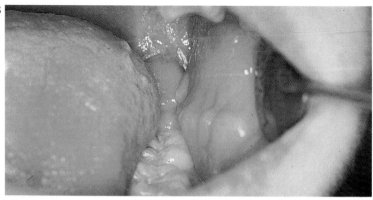

108 The buccal mucosa of a 15-year-old boy who complained of a swollen lower lip.
(a) What might these lesions be?
(b) What initial investigation should be carried out?
(c) What findings would be significant?
(d) What further investigations are indicated?
(e) Is the age of the patient significant?

109 A middle-aged patient complained of post-nasal discharge.
(a) What is the obvious sign?
(b) What is the value of this viewpoint?
(c) What other viewpoint may give equally useful information?
(d) What is the most significant possible diagnosis?

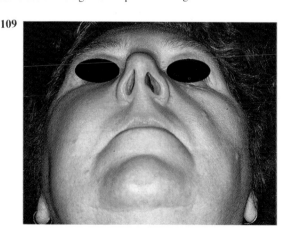

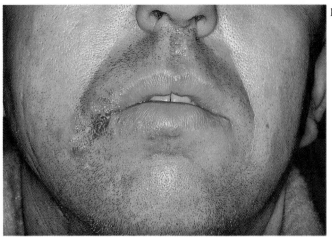

110 These lesions appeared after the extraction of a lower molar under local anaesthetic.
(a) What might they be?
(b) What is their relationship to the extraction?
(c) What should be done?

111 The patient has hypertrichosis and an oral abnormality.
(a) What is the condition?
(b) With what other generalised conditions may it be associated?
(c) What is its hereditary basis?

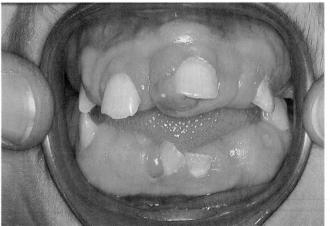

111

112

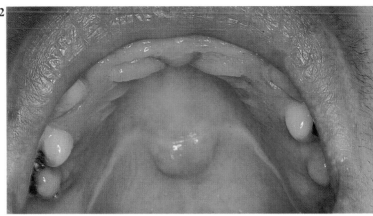

112 (a) What is the hard bony lump in the palate?
(b) What is its generalised significance?
(c) What action is recommended?
(d) What soft tissue lesion resembles it in appearance and site?

113 A middle-aged female complained of recurrent blistering of the gingivae.
(a) What might this be?
(b) How is the diagnosis confirmed?
(c) What other lesions should be suspected?

113

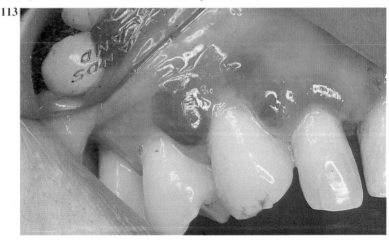

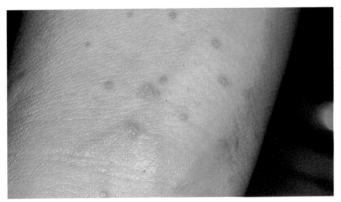

114 These lesions appeared on the wrist of a female with erosive oral lesions.
(a) What are they?
(b) Is the association with mouth lesions usual?
(c) What other sites may be involved?
(d) Are the skin lesions likely to last for a longer or shorter time than the oral lesion?

115 The appearance of this 12-year-old boy is similar to other members of his family.
(a) What is abnormal?
(b) With what is it associated?
(c) What is its genetic basis?
(d) What dental abnormality may be found?

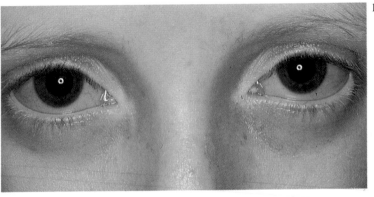

116

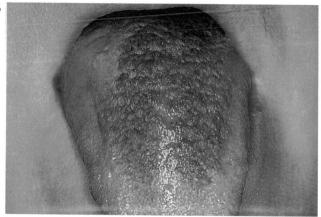

116 Recently this middle-aged patient had a course of antibiotic treatment for a chest infection.
(a) What is the oral condition?
(b) What is its relation to the history?
(c) What treatment is available?
(d) What is the origin of the brown coloration?

117 An irritable perioral lesion in a middle-aged female with a history of atopic diseases, including asthma and eczema.
(a) What might it be?
(b) What is the treatment?
(c) What is unusual about the treatment?

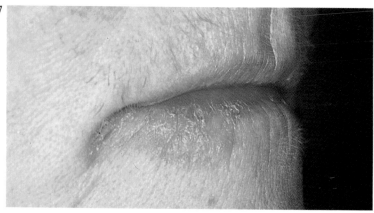

117

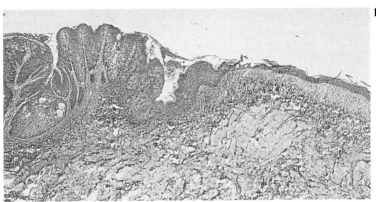

118 A biopsy taken from the buccal mucosa of a female with histologically proven lichen planus present for eight years.
(a) What does the section indicate?
(b) Is this common?
(c) In what particular form of lichen planus is it likely to occur most commonly?

119 The patient has a long history of recurrent oral ulceration classified as major aphthous ulceration.
(a) What are its characteristics?
(b) Is the morphology of the ulcer typical?
(c) With what may this form of ulceration be associated?
(d) What effective treatment is available?

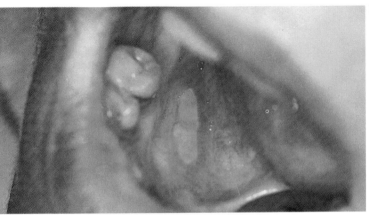

120

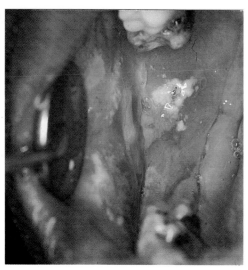

120 Erythema multiforme has been treated with antibiotic-steroid mouthwashes. The mouth initially responded well to the treatment but suddenly became sore again.
(a) What is the condition?
(b) What is its cause?
(c) What is the treatment?
(d) How can it be avoided?

121

121 Coxsackie A4 virus was cultured from these lesions.
(a) What might this be?
(b) What is the common age range of these patients?
(c) Normally how severe are the generalised symptoms?
(d) What other orofacial structure is involved occasionally?
(e) What other condition which produces oral vesicles may be associated with virus?

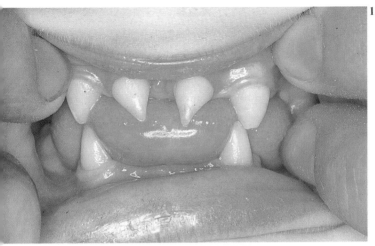

122 (a) What is the significance of the tooth morphology in this 14-year-old?
b) With what generalised conditions may it be associated?
c) Which tooth is most commonly thus formed in an otherwise normal dentition?

123 (a) What might be this painless condition of the buccal mucosa?
b) Why might its recognition be associated with a stomatitis?
c) What is its differential diagnostic importance?

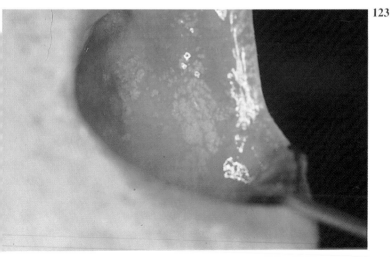

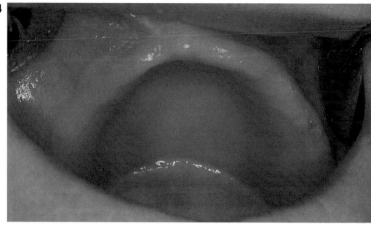

124 The oral condition is instantly recognisable.
(a) What is it?
(b) What is its origin?
(c) What is the more common name and why is it an inappropriate one?
(d) What generalised disease process should be suspected?

125 Dentures are not worn by this patient.
(a) What is the lesion on the alveolar crest?
(b) Is it potentially dangerous?
(c) What action is advisable?

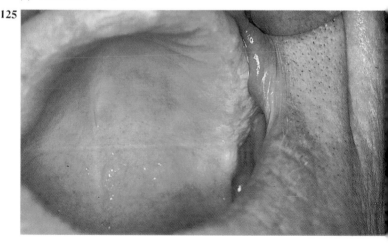

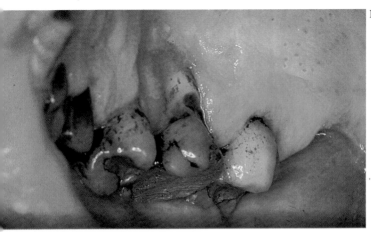

126, 127 This diabetic patient is a heavy pipe smoker.
(a) What is the condition in **126** which is relevant to the history?
(b) Is it considered to have malignant potential?
(c) What superimposed condition is in **127**?
(d) What investigations should be carried out?

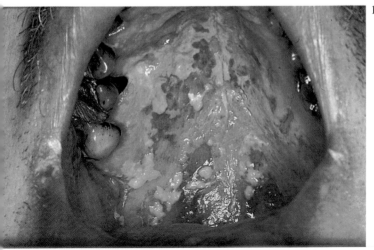

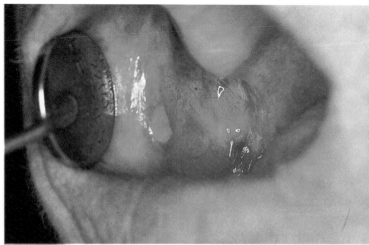

128, 129 Skin and oral lesions developed at about the same time in this middle-aged patient.
(a) What initial clinical differential diagnoses should be considered?
(b) What techniques would establish the diagnosis?
(c) What is the important prognostic factor in the differential diagnosis?
(d) What is the importance of accurate diagnosis of oral lesions in such conditions?

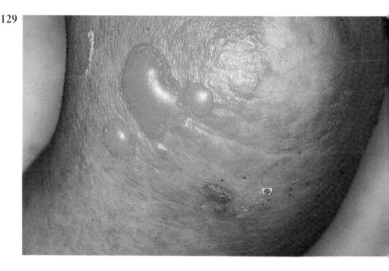

130 (a) What might be this painless lesion on the tongue?
(b) What is its usual location?
(c) Is there a significant age or sex distribution?

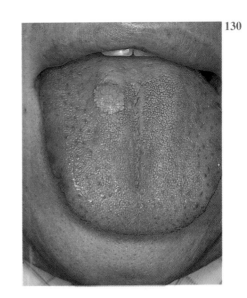

131 This mucosal abnormality appeared in a middle-aged patient.
(a) What is it?
(b) With what group of generalised disease processes may it be associated?
(c) What other mucosal abnormality may be associated?
(d) May a drug reaction be suspected?
(e) What similar appearance may follow a relatively common condition of the oral mucosa?

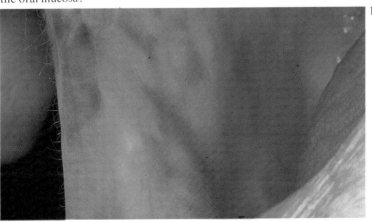

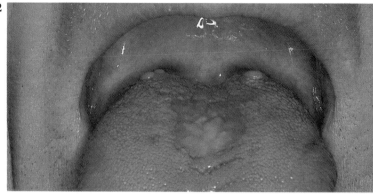

132 (a) What is this painless lesion of the tongue?
(b) What theory (now disproved) had previously explained its origin?
(c) What is now considered the origin of such a lesion?
(d) What action should be taken?

133 For many years this patient has been endentulous.
(a) What is the lesion?
(b) What factors contribute to its formation?
(c) Of what symptoms might the patient complain?
(d) What is a commonly associated oral lesion?
(e) What is the approach to treatment?

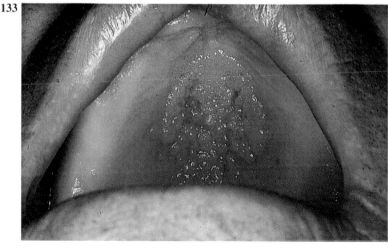

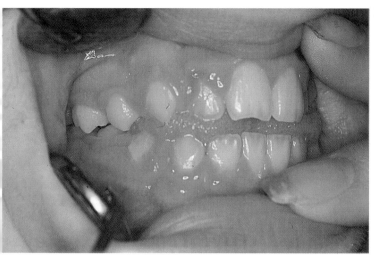

134 No systemic abnormality was found in this 12-year-old girl who had recently developed a rather proliferative gingivitis.
(a) What might it be?
(b) What is the mechanism involved?
(c) What is its relative incidence between males and females?
(d) What is the approach to treatment?

135 'Blood blisters' appeared suddenly on the palate during meals in this middle-aged lady. Full haematological screening tests showed no abnormality.
(a) What might it be?
(b) What conditions will be considered in a differential diagnosis?
(c) What investigations should be carried out?
(d) How should it be managed?

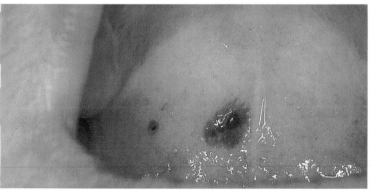

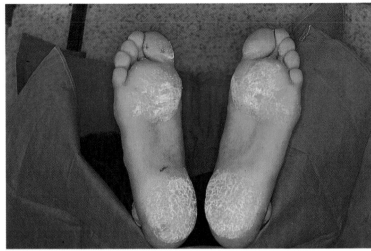

136 (a) What is the condition in the feet of this 30-year-old man?
(b) With what oral abnormality is it most commonly associated?
(c) With what periodontal abnormality may it be associated?
(d) With what oral and oesophageal abnormalities may it be associated?
(e) What is the genetic structure?

137 A lateral skull radiograph of a patient with symptoms suggestive of temporo-mandibular joint disorder.
(a) What is the most significant abnormal radiographic appearance?
(b) What radiographic appearance of the facial bone structures is consistent with this (although not diagnostic of any specific condition)?
(c) What is the diagnosis?
(d) What clinical signs and symptoms should be looked for?

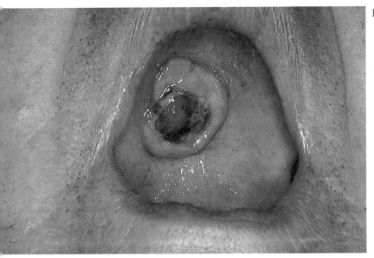

138, 139 Two superficially similar lesions are of quite different origin. **138** was slow-growing and painless while **139** was of rapid onset and very painful. In **139** a nearby molar tooth was tender to percussion.
(a) What clinical diagnoses should be considered in each case?
(b) What action should be taken in **138**?
(c) What is the initial action in **139**?

139

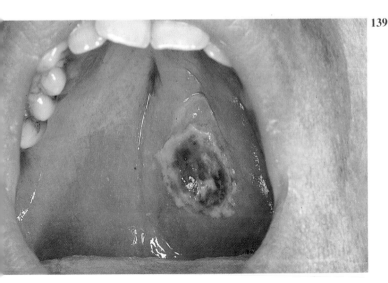

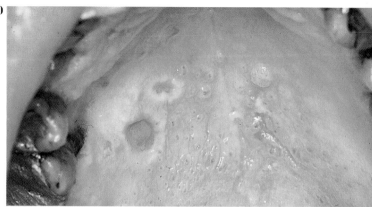

140 A middle-aged man has a clinically recognisable condition.
(a) What is it?
(b) What is the prognosis?
(c) What treatment might be effective?

141 The painless lesion in this 10-year-old boy has been present for at least four years.
(a) What is it?
(b) What is its nature?
(c) Is it a common site?
(d) Is the age of the patient characteristic?

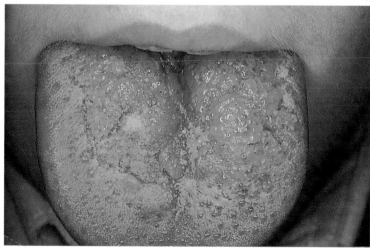

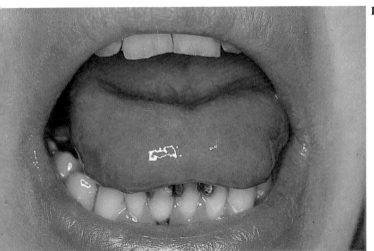

142 A 25-year-old male suffers from Addison's disease, hypoparathyroidism and pernicious anaemia. His tongue is intermittently sore.
(a) What is affecting the tongue?
(b) What other abnormality of the oral mucosa may occur?
(c) What is its relation to the patient's generalised diseases?
(d) What is the relationship between the generalised diseases themselves?

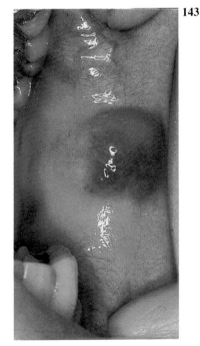

143 (a) What might be this common lesion of the oral mucosa?
(b) What is the cause?
(c) What is the effective causative factor?
(d) What other clinical diagnosis might be considered?

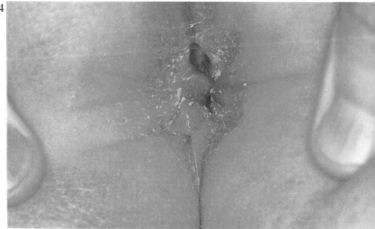

144 This is the perianal region of a 10-year-old boy with swelling of the lips and angular cheilitis.
(a) What may be the association?
(b) What investigations are called for?
(d) Of what anal symptoms might the patient complain?
(d) What element of treatment is common to both sites?

145 (a) What might be the condition in this 30-year-old pregnant lady?
(b) What causes this situation?
(c) What is the probable histology of the larger lesion in the molar area?
(d) What should be done about the localised lesion?
(e) What is the treatment for the more diffuse gingivitis?
(f) What is the likely long-term effect?

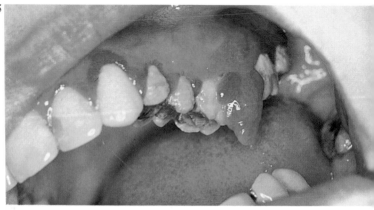

146, 147 These lesions are representative of a number of long-lasting ulcers on the oral mucosa, the nasal cavity and the skin of a 30-year-old man. Histology showed them to be vasculitic in origin and there was a marked proteinuria. He felt ill and debilitated.

(a) What should be suspected?

(b) What other oral manifestation might occur?

(c) What is the likely age and sex of such patients?

(d) What treatment is available?

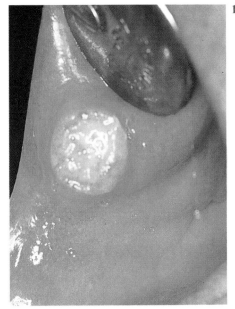

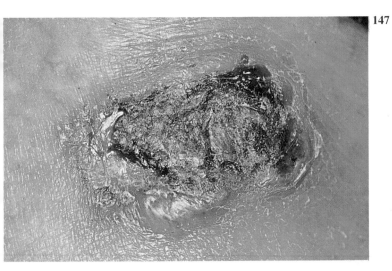

148

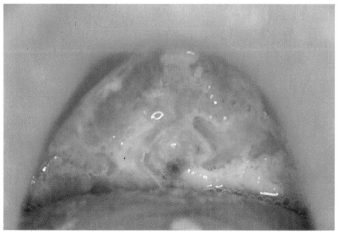

148 A renal transplant patient is under treatment by very high doses of steroids, during an episode of rejection. Candidiasis has been diagnosed but the lesions have not responded to antifungal treatment.
(a) What might these lesions be?
(b) What investigations should be carried out?
(c) What is the basis of treatment?

149

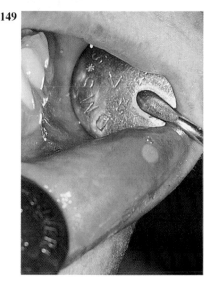

149 There were depressed serum and red cell folate levels in this 20-year-old female.
(a) What is the condition?
(b) What may cause the lowered serum levels?
(c) What is the significant difference between the two indices?
(d) What might be the connection of the oral lesion with the abnormal folate levels?
(e) What generalised condition might be associated with the two factors?
(f) What further investigation might be considered?
(g) What treatment might be contemplated?

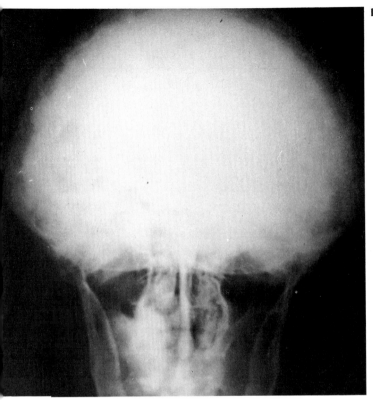

150 The patient complained of poorly fitting dentures and of ill-defined but severe facial pain.
(a) What does the radiograph suggest?
(b) What initial biochemical tests should be conducted?
(c) What is the origin of the pain?

151 (a) What is this extremely painful facial rash?
(b) What is the long-term sequel?
(c) What action should be taken?
(d) In what group of generalised diseases may there be a high incidence?

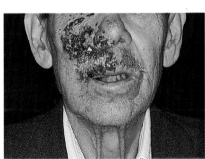

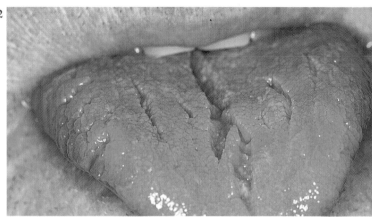

152 The tongue of this adult man is symptom-free.
(a) What might be the origin of the fissures?
(b) What is their clinical significance?
(c) In what circumstances may such fissures become painful?
(d) In what pathological conditions may the pattern of fissuring be modified?
(e) What minimal feature shown might be significant in slightly altered circumstances?

153 A virtually pain-free but long-lasting lesion of the tongue in a middle-aged male with active ulcerative colitis.
(a) What might it be?
(b) Where may similar lesions appear?
(c) What more aggressive oral lesions may appear in ulcerative colitis?

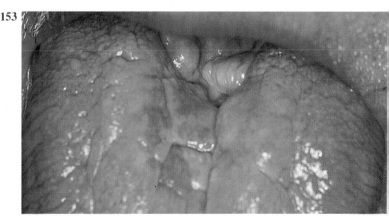

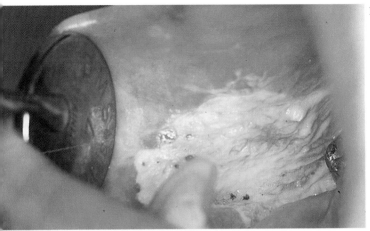

154 This is a painless lesion in a middle-aged female.
 a) What is the clinical diagnosis?
 b) What initial steps should be taken?
 c) What definitive treatment might be considered?

155 There is gingival soreness and fragility in this middle-aged woman. A gingival biopsy was unhelpful, but a biopsy taken from the mucosa of the sulcus showed linear deposits of IgG and C3 at the basal zone on immunofluorescent study.
 a) What might be the clinical diagnosis?
 b) Why would the gingival biopsy be unhelpful?
 c) What diagnosis is suggested by the immunofluorescence results?
 d) What alternative diagnosis might be considered on clinical grounds?

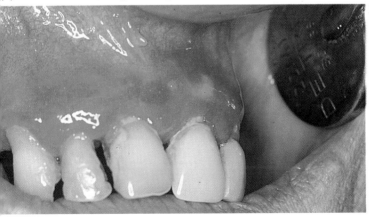

156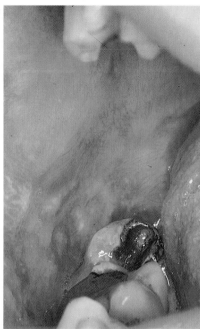

156 A slightly painful lesion of the buccal mucosa of a middle-aged man.

(a) What initial clinical diagnoses should be considered?

(b) What steps should be taken to determine further action?

(c) What form might treatment take?

(d) What might be the significance of the red area of mucosa?

157 A 20-year-old man has recurrent episodic scaling of his lips. Tissue examined shows that keratin and parakeratin is being exfoliated.

(a) What is the condition?

(b) With what is it associated?

(c) What is the treatment?

157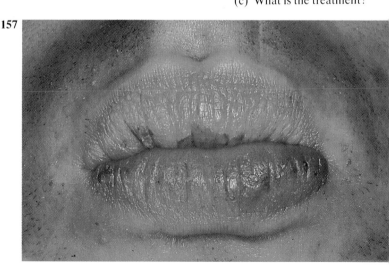

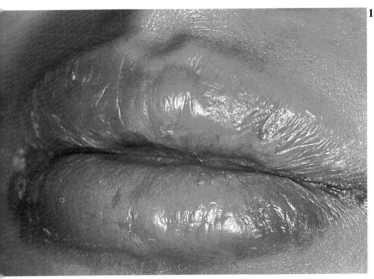

158, 159 A 20-year-old girl had developed a lesion of facial herpes 10 days before the onset of these lesions.
a) What is the diagnosis?
b) What is unusual about the clinical presentation?
c) What treatment should be considered?
d) What is the long-term prognosis?
e) What is the long-term management?

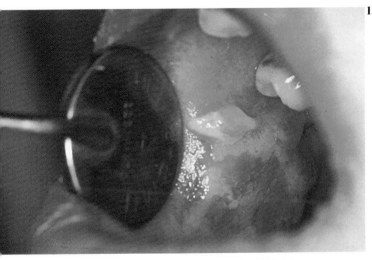

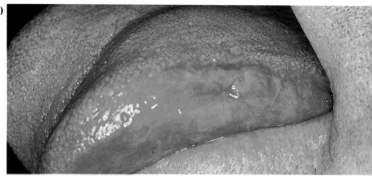

160 A 60-year-old male presented with a slightly sore lesion of the tongue, partial anaesthesia of the right trigeminal nerve and muscular weakness.
(a) What type of condition might be involved?
(b) What initial action should be taken?
(c) What further investigations should be conducted?
(d) What form of therapy might be considered?

161 This long-lasting lesion on the tongue of a 25-year-old man causes occasional mild irritation and infrequent bleeding from the area.
(a) What is it?
(b) Such a lesion occasionally may be of a more complex kind. What is the complexity?
(c) What action should be taken?

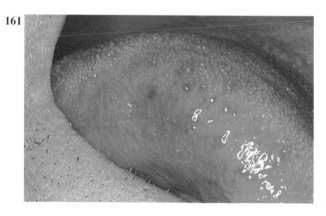

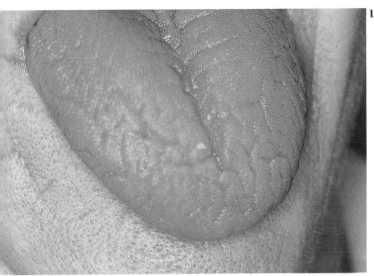

162, 163 A 40-year-old female has systemic lupus erythematosus.
(a) What complication is shown?
(b) What immunological changes are likely to be demonstrated on investigation?
(c) What is the significance of the personal details?
(d) What action should be taken in respect of the oral problem?

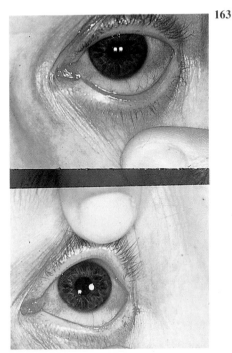

164

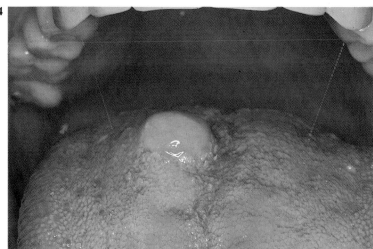

164 (a) What might be this solitary painless lesion of unknown duration?
(b) What significant condition is it unlikely to be?
(c) What action should be taken?

165

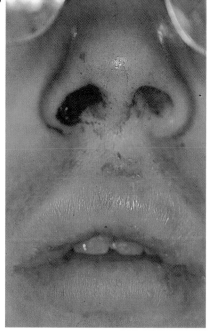

165 A 20-year-old male is suffering a recurrent attack of erythema multiforme although the oral lesions are minimal.
(a) What is the condition illustrated?
(b) What is its origin?
(c) In what other conditions may a similar situation occur?

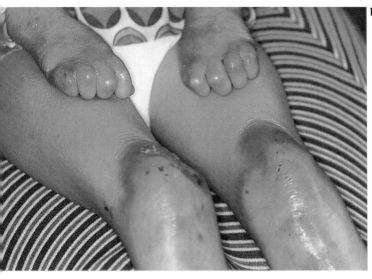

166, **167** The young patient has a genetically determined skin disease with oral repercussions.
(a) What is it?
(b) What are its generalised manifestations?
(c) What are the oral problems involved?
(d) What are the difficulties involved in dental treatment?

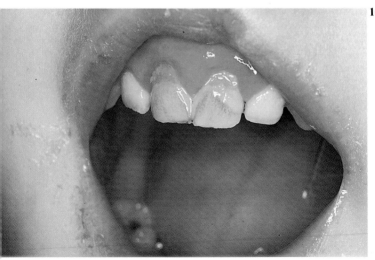

168

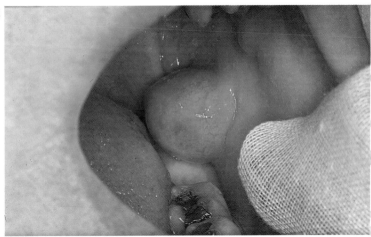

168 (a) What might be this painless lesion of several years' standing?
(b) What alternative diagnoses should be considered?
(c) What action should be taken?
(d) What controversy exists as to the nomenclature of lesions of this kind?

169 The tongue is irritated by chocolate or cheese.
(a) What might be the lesion?
(b) What is the significance of these foodstuffs?
(c) What is to be done?

169

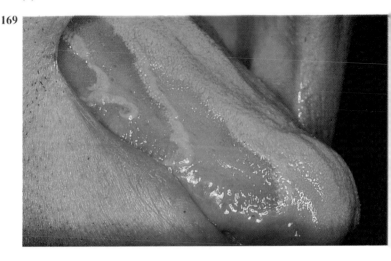

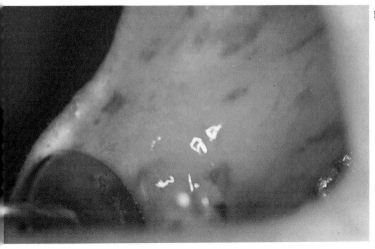

170 (a) What is visible in this healthy middle-aged patient?
(b) What systemic factors should be eliminated?
(c) In the absence of any systemic factors how might this be described?
(d) What cytological abnormality might be found?

171 A painless lesion on the buccal mucosa of a 15-year-old girl.
(a) What might it be?
(b) What is the prognosis?
(c) What action should be taken?

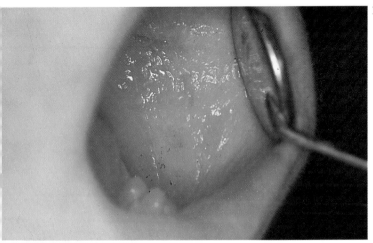

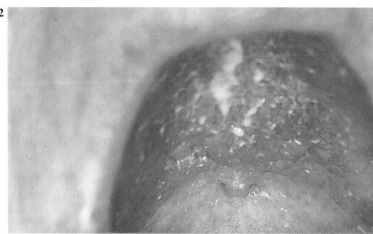

172, 173 Addison's disease (hypopadrenocorticism) is under control by corticosteroid therapy.
(a) What is the condition shown?
(b) What is the fundamental problem which results in this oral condition?
(c) Why is the oral condition not under control as is the generalised one?
(d) What is the lesion in **173** likely to be?
(e) What is the approach to treatment?

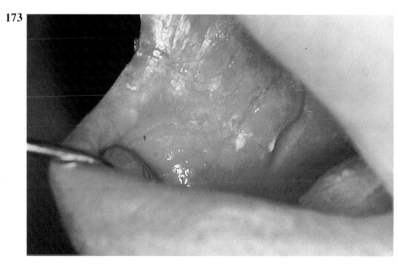

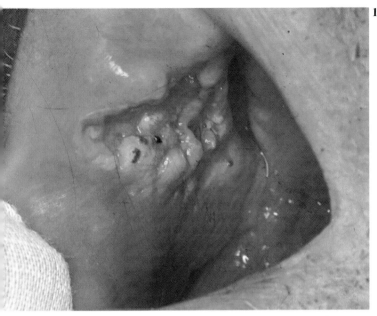

174 (a) What is this lesion in a middle-aged male?
(b) Is this a common site?
(c) Is there commonly a pre-cursor lesion?
(d) What is the prognosis?

175 A fluid-filled lesion on the under surface of the tongue of some months' duration.
(a) What might it be?
(b) What is unusual about it?

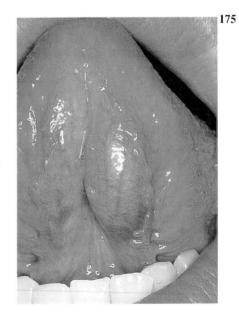

176

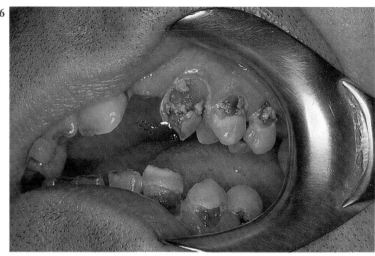

176, 177 These two patients have undergone radiotherapy, **176** for carcinoma in the tonsilar area, **177** for carcinoma of the lower lip.
(a) What is the change in **176**?
(b) What is its cause?
(c) What can be done to minimise it?
(d) What is the change in **177**?
(e) What eventual problems might develop?

177

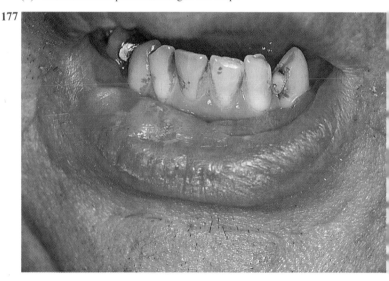

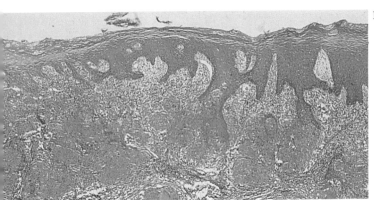

178 A section of a biopsy taken from a buccal lesion in a patient with a history of exposure to tuberculosis.
(a) What does the histology suggest?
(b) How would you establish the diagnosis?
(c) What further clinical investigations are essential?
(d) What form of treatment should be contemplated?

179 A middle-aged lady has had intermittent swelling of the lower lip over some years. It is now virtually permanent. She has had four episodes of transient facial nerve weakness and suffers from migraine type headaches.
(a) What is this?
(b) What other sign might be expected?
(c) What may be found on biopsy of the buccal mucosa?
(d) What is its genetic basis?
(e) What other conditions should be considered in the initial differential diagnosis?

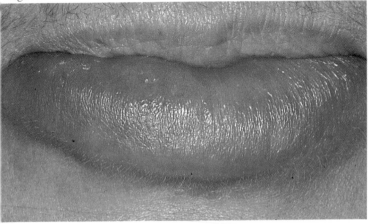

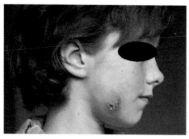

180 A persistent discharging sinus on the cheek of a young female.
(a) What might it be?
(b) What investigations are necessary?
(c) What is the approach to treatment?

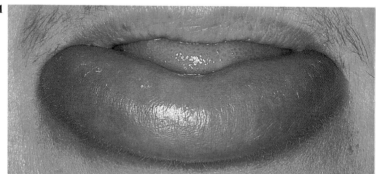

181 A female had a long history of painless soft tissue swellings of rapid onset, predominantly about the face; no local cause could be found. There was a similar family history with instances of respiratory embarrassment.
(a) What might this be?
(b) What investigations should be carried out?
(c) What steps should be taken?

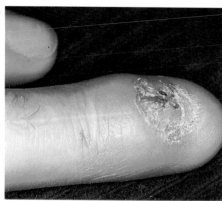

182 For most of his life a 25-year-old patient has had recurrent oral candidiasis.
(a) What is the connection between the mouth and the finger-nail abnormality?
(b) What generalised disease process may be responsible?
(c) What treatment might be effective?
(d) What immunological abnormalities might be expected?

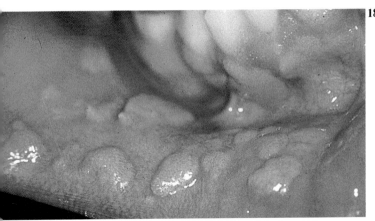

183 A young South African coloured man developed these symptom-free lesions of the labial and buccal mucosa.
a) What are they?
b) What will the histology show?
c) What is their aetiology?
d) What differential diagnosis might be considered on appearance alone?
e) What is the significance of the personal history?
f) What treatment should be used?
g) What is the prognosis?

184 (a) What is the gingivitis in a patient with Crohn's disease?
(b) What is its histology?
(c) What is its treatment?

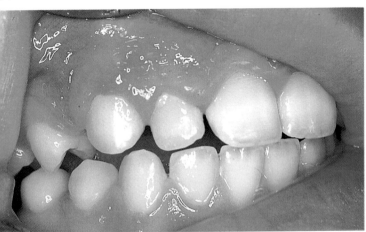

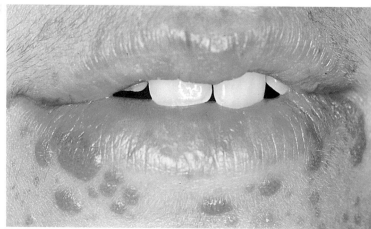

185 An 18-year-old girl developed painless perioral lesions. Biopsy showed non-caseating tuberculoid structure; the only other abnormality was enlargement of hilar lymph nodes on chest X-ray. Kveim test positive.
(a) What might this be?
(b) Is this a common presentation?
(c) How is the Kveim test carried out?
(d) What is the treatment for these lesions?
(e) What is the prognosis?

186 A renal transplant patient on high dosage steroid therapy to combat rejection developed this lesion.
(a) What might it be?
(b) Is it significant?
(c) What steps should be taken?

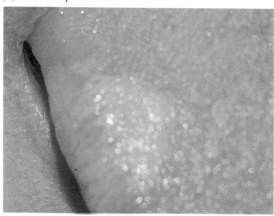

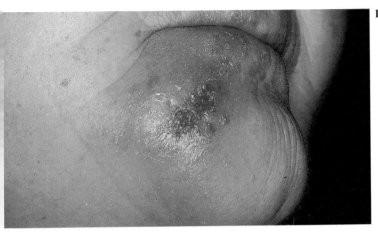

187 (a) What is the lesion in this middle-aged patient with chronic lymphocytic leukaemia?
(b) What is the precipitating factor in this case?
(c) What steps should be taken?

188 A 65-year-old patient has new dentures after 25 years. He is complaining of a sore tongue.
(a) What might be this condition?
(b) What investigations should be carried out?
(c) What action should be taken?

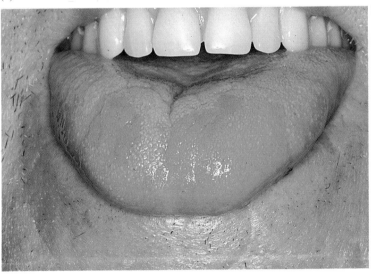

189

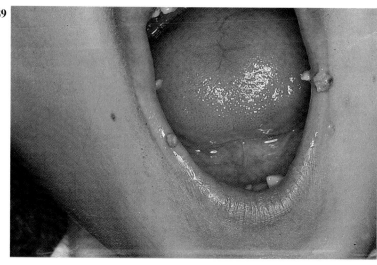

189, 190 (a) What are the related lesions in this 10-year-old boy?
(b) What is the method of transmission?
(c) What action should be taken?

190

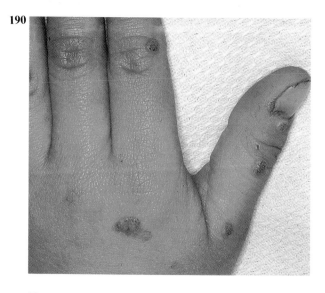

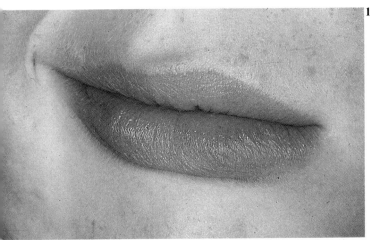

191 A 12-year-old boy developed this abnormality within the last three days. He is attempting to smile.
a) What might it be?
b) What initial simple neurological test should be carried out?
c) What other symptoms might be present?
d) What action should be taken?

192 A 12-year-old girl with a genetic susceptibility to oral leukoplakia (see **52, 53**).
a) What is the term applied to such a lesion?
b) What is its prognosis?
c) What action should be taken?

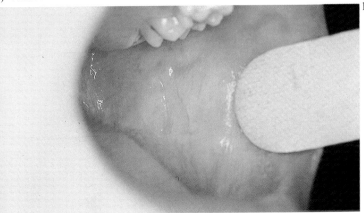

193

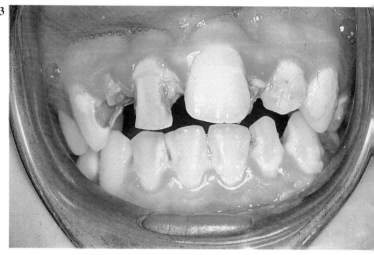

193 This patient has juvenile onset diabetes mellitus.
(a) What is the relationship between the generalised and dental conditions?
(b) What steps should be taken?
(c) What other oral complications may occur?

194

194 A painless lesion of the buccal mucosa in a 60-year-old male smoker.
(a) What might it be?
(b) The clinical appearance supports one particular clinical diagnosis. What is it?
(c) What is the significance of the personal details?
(d) What action should be taken?

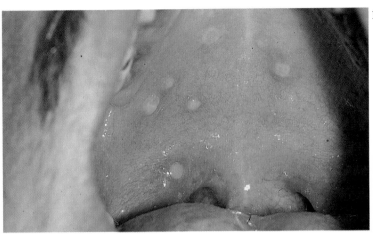

195 A painful vesicular lesion developed on the palate of this 20-year-old. Herpes simplex 2 virus was demonstrated in swabs from the lesions.
(a) What is unusual about this situation?
(b) What other viral aetiology might have been considered in a clinical diagnosis?
(c) What is the significance of the identification of herpes 2 virus?

196 A 60-year-old female presented with this lesion.
(a) What is the most likely diagnosis?
(b) What action should be taken?
(c) What is the prognosis?
(d) What is the significance of the personal details?

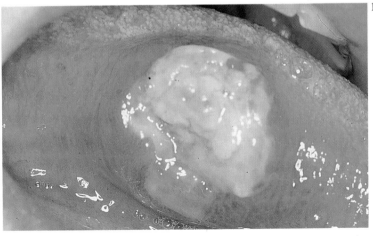

197

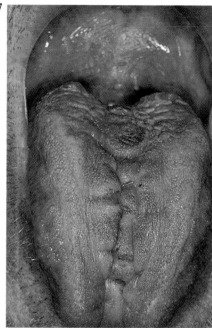

197 This patient has been under treatment for four days with local steroid and antibiotic mouthwashes. The tongue condition developed over the period of treatment.
(a) What is the condition?
(b) What is to be done?
(c) What prophylactic measures can be taken to avoid it?

198 (a) To what extent does this man's poor periodontal condition relate to his Indian origin?
(b) What is the significant aetiological factor in the clinical picture?

198

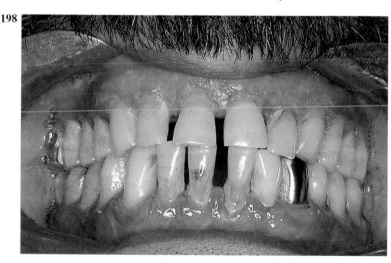

199 (a) What may be the relationship of this patient's psoriasis to the abnormality of the tongue?
(b) What other oral lesions have been described in psoriasis?
(c) What other oro-facial problems may arise?

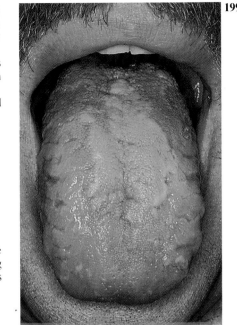

200 These oral lesions have developed recently in a young female with systemic lupus erythematosus.
(a) What might they be?
(b) What is their cause?
(c) What other oral lesions may appear?
(d) What is the significance of the personal details?

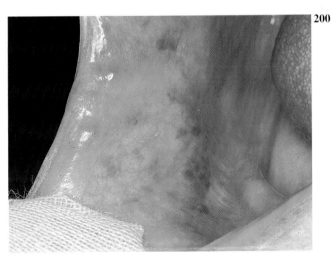

ANSWERS

1 (a) Lichen planus.
(b) Erosive lesions may occur as well as non-erosive lesions with a wide morpho logical range, some of which may simulate other conditions.
(c) None but it is, in general, symptom free.
(d) None has been established. A relation with maturity onset diabetes and with hypertension has not been clearly proven. Lichen planus may appear as a response to a wide range of drug therapy – the so-called lichenoid reaction.
(e) A few cases of malignancy occurring in established lichen planus have been reported, most of which have been in erosive lesions. In view of the many patients with oral lichen planus, the incidence must be less than one per cent.

2 (a) Acid erosion.
(b) There is an unusually acid environment – either due to increased input of acidic foods or drinks or to persistent vomiting. Often there is an excessive input of fruit or fruit drinks as part of a slimming diet. There is also often an element of excessive abrasion involved.
(c) Any condition in which regular vomiting may occur – in this case, the bulimic variant of anorexia nervosa was responsible.

3 (a) A typical floor mouth leukoplakia with the so-called ebbing tide appearance.
(b) It is essential to take a biopsy to determine the degree of epithelial atypia. Further action depends entirely upon the histological appearance and may include surgical excision, laser or cryosurgery or, simply, long-term observation.
(c) Previously thought to be relatively innocuous, it has now been demonstrated that there is a considerable premalignant potential in these lesions.

4 (a) There is a wide range of possibilities, but a salivary gland neoplasm is high in the list of differential diagnoses.
(b) The nature of the lesion should be established by biopsy with facilities available for immediate definitive surgery.

5, 6 (a) An external sinus draining from a periapical lesion on one of the carious teeth present.
(b) X-ray normally shows the origin of the sinus – this may be an unsuspected buried root in an otherwise edentulous mouth.
(c) Extraction of the tooth or root involved. If the sinus does not disappear curettage or excision of the sinus tract may be necessary.

7 (a) A gumma (a tertiary syphilitic lesion).
(b) Serological tests for syphilis. If there is doubt a biopsy should be taken from the edge of the lesion (a neoplasm is a further possible diagnosis).
(c) Even in older patients with otherwise apparently inactive long-standing syphilis antibiotic treatment may result in a generalised improvement in health.

8 (a) Actinic cheilitis.
(b) The effect of constant exposure to the sun is thought to be highly significant in the formation of this lesion which is far more common in male than in female patients.
(c) It has a high potential for malignant transformation (the term 'lip at risk' is often used to describe it).

9 (a) It was present throughout the whole period of the formation of the crowns of the teeth.
(b) Fluorosis – the patient was born and lived in a region with an extremely high fluoride concentration in the water supply (>10p.p.m.).

(c) No. Teeth of this kind, although with deficiencies in the enamel, are relatively resistant to caries.

(d) Fluorosis affects the deciduous teeth much less severely than the permanent teeth. It is thought that there is a partially effective placental barrier against the fluoride.

10 (a) Bleeding diatheses, bullous mucosal lesions such as pemphigoid and the apparently spontaneous 'idiopathic blood blister' formation should be considered. The oral lesions of pemphigoid, although usually filled with clear fluid, often contain bloodstained fluid because of secondary bleeding from the base of the bulla. This patient was showing early manifestations of thrombocytopoenia.

(b) A full range of haematology screening tests to eliminate a bleeding disorder and biopsy (of an intact bulla if possible) with immunofluorescent studies.

(c) In the absence of any reversible clotting disorder the prevention of blister formation is very difficult. In established pemphigoid, local steroid applications (by aerosol) may be effective.

11 (a) Monostotic fibrous dysplasia.

(b) Serum calcium, phosphorous and alkaline phosphatase levels are normal. However, in patients of this age the alkaline phosphatase levels are much higher than in the normal adult and may be difficult to interpret.

(c) Treatment is conservative – the lesions generally become static in early adult life and cosmetic recontouring can then be carried out.

12 (a) Crohn's disease.

(b) Proliferative lesions of the oral mucosa containing non-caseating tuberculoid granulomas.

(c) Biopsy of an oral granuloma, nutritional screening and contrast radiography initially. Further endoscopy etc may then be indicated.

(d) Oral Chrohn's disease may accompany or precede more widespread gastro-intestinal changes. In some patients the condition appears to be restricted to the mouth although it must never be assumed that this will continue.

13 (a) Leukaemia – in this case, acute myeloid leukaemia.

(b) A full blood count (including platelets) is essential.

(c) Pregnancy gingivitis, in its early stages, would be an obvious consideration although the relatively pink (rather than red) colour of the gingivae is against this.

14 (a) This is the characteristic histological appearance of an adenocystic carcinoma ('cylindroma' in an older terminology).

(b) It is an insidious lesion which has a bad reputation for local and widespread dissemination, often after a long period of time.

(c) Immediate arrangements for effective surgery should be made. The possibility of metasteses (especially to the lung) should be borne in mind. Long term review, even after apparently successful surgery, should be carried out.

15 (a) Submucous fibrosis.

(b) The condition remains a mystery. Almost entirely confined to patients from the Indian subcontinent and nearby areas, its cause is unknown.

(c) No known effective treatment.

16 (a) A lichenoid reaction to an anti-rheumatic drug. Such reactions are relatively common and may involve almost any of the drugs in general use.

(b) Biopsy of a non-ulcerated area usually shows a histological picture similar to that of lichen planus.

(c) Withdrawal of the drug involved is the first obvious step. However, the response may be much less immediate than expected – lichenoid reactions of this kind may take a long time to settle, even when aided by the therapy which would be used for non drug-induced lichen planus.

17 (a) Patients may become B12 and iron deficient following gastrectomy; a restricted diet may also lead to folate deficiency. This patient suffered from all three of these. Angular cheilitis with an element of candidal leukoplakia often follows, as shown.

(b) A full haematological screen is essential. Swabs should be taken to identify the predominant organisms present – candida and staphylococci are the most likely. If the leukoplakia is a dominant feature, then assessment by biopsy is also indicated.

(c) Replacement therapy as indicated by the screening tests, local treatment by antifungals/antibiotics according to the bacteriology report and, if eventually felt necessary, treatment as for commissural leukoplakia – perhaps by cryosurgery.

18 (a) Chronic candidiasis – patients with myasthenia gravis and related conditions have impaired immune function (particularly affecting T cell activity).

(b) Haematological abnormalities are common.

(c) Topical antifungals – currently, the imidazoles are the most satisfactory.

19 (a) A submandibular gland.

(b) Dilatation of the submandibular duct.

(c) Long-standing obstruction of the submandibular duct – this might be completely painless. The initial causative factor might be calculus (perhaps in an early 'non-calcified' phase or having been expelled). The radiopaque area in the anterior part of the duct is not a calculus but a globule of contrast medium.

20 (a) Squamous cell carcinoma.

(b) Carcinoma of the lower lip occurs predominantly in older male patients.

(c) This site is one which is most responsive to treatment – either by relatively limited surgery or by radiotherapy. A simple surgical approach is often curative.

21 (a) The so called 'pink spot'. It is the result of internal resorption of the hard tissues of the tooth by abnormal pulpal activity. In this case a small external perforation has occurred.

(b) The precise aetiology is not known but trauma to the tooth is thought to be a major factor.

(c) Evidently the tooth has been traumatised and there is a coronal fracture.

22 (a) An eruption cyst – a cyst lying superficial to the crown of an erupting tooth.

(b) Unless there is interference with the occlusion, the cyst may be left to rupture spontaneously. If it persists, or becomes troublesome because of interference with the occlusion, a simple incision may be carried out.

(c) The cyst wall is covered by epithelium on both sides of a thin connective tissue layer – on the oral surface by oral epithelium and on the inner surface by non keratinising squamous epithelium of odontogenic origin.

23 (a) Transposition of the left maxillary incisors.

(b) Generally, this is an isolated phenomenon but in a few cases is present in patients with abnormalities in the number of teeth (either missing or supernumerary teeth).

(c) There are no reports of transposition occurring in the primary dentition as such although, in some cases of multiple abnormality, retained primary teeth may be involved and appear in a 'transposed' site.

24 (a) A typical 'speckled leukoplakia' in a characteristic site.

(b) They are reported as having a much higher incidence of malignant transformation than from homogenous leukoplakias.

(c) Histological assessment is essential. If, as is likely, infestation by candida is found, preliminary treatment by antifungals may reduce both the extent and apparent aggressiveness of the lesion. Definitive treatment should follow – cryosurgery is often very useful.

5 (a) The focal distribution of lymphocytes.
b) It virtually never occurs in lichen planus and, if seen, should be an immediate warning of the possible diagnosis of some form of connective tissue disease. These oral lesions may resemble closely those of lichen planus.
c) A full range of immunological investigations with particular reference to the presence of auto-antibodies. The patient should be assessed (even in the absence of obvious symptoms) by a physician experienced in the field of connective tissue disease.

6 (a) Recurrent oral herpes simplex.
b) Very uncommon. The lack of distressing symptoms is characteristic. Severe attacks of recurrent oral herpes resembling primary herpetic stomatitis virtually never occur in the normal patient but may occur in highly immunosuppressed and otherwise compromised patients.
c) A full immunological and haematology work up. However, in the few patients of this kind seen by the author, no fundamental abnormality has been found.

7, 28 (a) Hand-foot-mouth disease. Similar lesions were found on his feet.
b) Coxsackie virus (most commonly type A16).
c) Isolation of the virus – faecal specimens are most productive of viral particles if vesicle fluid cannot be obtained.
d) None. The condition is practically always mild and self-limiting.

9 (a) Development of eye lesions in these circumstances strongly suggests Behçet's syndrome. They are usually the result of a uveitis – not of corneal ulceration.
b) Specialist ophthalmological opinion is highly desirable. Management is usually with relatively high doses of steroids.
c) HLA B5 may be a marker of Behçet's syndrome with ocular involvement and B12 of the mucocutaneous type. However, the evidence is not firm.

0 (a) Geographic tongue (erythema migrans).
b) Unknown.
c) No generalised abnormality has been shown convincingly to be associated with this condition and screening tests are invariably non-productive.
c) No treatment is known.

1 (a) Angular cheilitis.
b) Unsatisfactory dentures (particularly if resulting in a reduced vertical dimension), anatomical deep folds at the angles, haematological abnormalities, generalised ill health and Crohn's disease.
c) Candida albicans and staphylococci.
d) Denture sore mouth (denture stomatitis).

2, 33 (a) A giant cell epullis.
b) Hyperparathyroidism. The majority of jaw lesions in this condition are central and are seen as osteolytic lesions on X-ray. However, peripheral giant cell lesions may also have this association.
c) Serum chemistry profiles.
d) Raised serum calcium and lowered serum phosphorus levels. Alkaline phosphatase levels are less significant.
e) Parathyroid adenoma.

4 (a) An intraepithelial bulla.
b) Pemphigus.
c) Immunofluorescent techniques to demonstrate the presence of antibody complexes in relation to the desmosomes of the stratum spinosum.
d) The oral lesions of pemphigus appear well before the skin lesions in a significant proportion of cases thus enabling early diagnosis.
e) There is a high proportion of Jewish patients among those with pemphigus.

35 (a) A herpetic whitlow – commonly contracted by dentists following contac with patients with active or latent herpetic infections.
(b) This can be a long lasting problem and should be treated vigorously with topica and systemic anti-viral agents.

36 (a) Acute herpetic stomatitis.
(b) No previous attacks of this kind or recurrent facial herpes.
(c) Rising titres of antibodies to Herpes simplex over ten days. Viral growth i tissue culture or direct electron microscopy of samples from the vesicular lesion will confirm the diagnosis more rapidly.
(d) An approximately 50 per cent chance of developing recurrent chronic facia herpes. Recurrent chronic intraoral herpes is very rare; recurrent acute herpeti stomatitis virtually unknown in healthy patients.

37 (a) Pemphigoid in one of its variants – if only the oral mucosa and the eye ar involved, mucosal pemphigoid is the likely eventual diagnosis.
(b) Oral lesions are usually noticed first but, on examination early eye lesions ma be found.
(c) Biopsy of an oral lesion (or of tissue nearby if only a ruptured bulla is available examined by immunofluorescent techniques.
(d) Deposition of IgG and C3 along the basal complex.

38 (a) A target lesion.
(b) Erythema multiforme.
(c) A wide range of drugs and also Herpes simplex infections. In most patients none are found.

39 (a) Gingival fibromatosis (idiopathic gingival hyperplasia).
(b) In a few patients, with hypertrichosis and, more rarely, with various birth defects.
(c) None.
(d) Conservative management as a localised dental problem.

40 (a) The P.A.S. positive structures are candidal pseudo-hyphae within the epithelium.
(b) Lesions of this kind (candida – leukoplakias) have a higher potential fo malignant transformation than those without a candidal component.
(c) Antifungal treatment might result in some recession of the lesion and make surgical management less difficult.

41 (a) Major erosive lichen planus.
(b) Areas of typical non-erosive lichen planus on other parts of the oral mucosa.
(c) Biopsy of a non-eroded area close to the lesion – this would likely show the changes of lichen planus.
(d) Most patients with this form of lichen planus are in the older age range (6C years +).

42 (a) The linear deposition of antibody at the basement zone is compatible with sub epithelial bulla formation.
(b) Pemphigoid.

43 (a) Arthritic erosion of the condyle heads.
(b) Residual deformity, or remodelling in less marked cases.
(c) Treatment as for the generalised condition. Local steroid injections have been advocated to supplement this. Appliances may be provided if the position become static.

44, 45 (a) Chronic discoid lupus.
(b) Lichen planus.
(c) It would resemble that of lichen planus except for a focal distribution of lymphocytes in the corium rather than a band-like distribution.
(d) Malignant transformation occurs in a small proportion of these lip lesions.

46 (a) Perioral dermatitis.
(b) It is much more common in young adult females than in others.
(c) Unknown although some cases have been reported following the use of steroid creams.
(d) Steroid treatment should be approached with great caution. Paradoxically some patients respond to 1 per cent hydrocortisone cream.

47 (a) A typical traumatic ulcer caused by an orthodontic appliance.
(b) Removal of the source of trauma and subsequent observation.

48 (a) In spite of its resemblance to herpes, this is a bacterial infective lesion.
(b) In the highly immunosuppressed patient amost any organism (including those normally considered as commensals).
(c) Identification and determination of antibiotic sensitivity of the organisms involved.
(d) The appropriate antibiotic should be used systemically and locally.

49 (a) Primary herpes.
(b) Leukaemia – in view of the rather hyperplastic gingivae.
(c) A full blood count and film survey.
(d) In viral infections abnormal white cells (particularly polymorphs).

50 (a) Loss of secretory units, ductal hyperplasia and lymphocytic infiltration – all as expected in Sjogren's syndrome.
(b) Connective tissue disease should be considered – rheumatoid arthritis being the most likely. The eyes should also be examined for the possibility of lachrimal gland degeneration.
(c) When associated with salivery gland degeneration it is effectively irreversible.

51 (a) Acute pseudomembranous candidiasis (thrush).
(b) Exaggerated gingivitis and dry mouth.
(c) Sialosis (non-inflammatory swelling).

52, 53 (a) Tylosis – hyperkeratosis of the soles of the feet (and the palms of the hands).
(b) In a small number of patients this is associated with oral leukoplakia and, in particular, keratotic changes in the gingivae.
(c) Carcinoma of the oesophagus can occur in small groups of related patients in association with tylosis and leukoplakia, as illustrated.
(d) Transmitted as a dominant characteristic of high penetrance.
(e) In the Papillon-Lefevre syndrome tylosis is associated with gross premature degeneration of the periodontium in both primary and secondary dentitions (see 135).

54 (a) An oral lesion treated by painting with gentian violet.
(b) No, gentian violet has great disadvantages over almost all other non-specific treatment.
(c) Hypersensitivity reactions have been reported.

55 (a) Swelling of the parotid gland.
(b) Dry mouth and dry eyes.
(c) Sjogren's syndrome.
(d) Parotid swelling secondary to arthritic involvement of the temporo-mandibular joint.

56 (a) Band-like hypoplastic enamel in the two upper central incisors with minor structural abnormalities in other teeth.
(b) Between birth and approximately one year.
(c) Although there may be no identifiable cause, some metabolic abnormality (however slight) must have been involved.

57, 58 (a) Both are variants if gingival lichen planus.

(b) It is most common in young and middle aged females.

(c) Biopsy using immunofluorescent techniques. Buccal lesions give a better biopsy specimen than the gingivae where secondary inflammatory changes are invariably present and make interpretation difficult.

(d) Pemphigoid.

(e) Desquamative gingivitis.

59 (a) Melanin deposition, amalgam pigmentation, haemangioma.

(b) X-ray for the presence of amalgam particles – although the metal may be widely distributed and non-opaque.

(c) If there is clear evidence of recent onset with no evidence of amalgam or of a haemangiomatous origin then melanoma must be suspected. Biopsy should be a wide and definitive excision.

60 (a) Erythema multiforme – the lower lip is often severely involved.

(b) The skin, the eyes and other mucous membranes.

(c) Young adults.

(d) The pattern of recurrence is individual to the patient with attacks three to six months. The condition usually subsides after two or three years.

(e) Local steroids and antibiotics if the mouth only is involved. If the condition is more generalised systemic steroids and antibiotics may be necessary.

61, 62 (a) Villous atrophy – as occurs in coeliac disease.

(b) Approximately 6 per cent of patients with recurrent oral ulceration have a flat jejunal mucosa on biopsy.

(c) None – it may be classified either as minor or major aphthous ulceration or herpetiform ulceration.

(d) Hypersensitivity to alpha gliaden, a constituent of gluten, present in wheat flour.

(e) If a gluten free diet is adhered to, the jejunal mucosa will revert to normal and the oral ulceration will go into remission.

63 (a) Punctate lichen planus.

(b) Candidiasis, Fordyces spots or speckled leukoplakia.

(c) Confirmation by biopsy followed by observation.

64 (a) A solitary lesion of geographic tongue.

(b) None, other than reassurance.

65 (a) Microdontia of the permanent dentition.

(b) Retained deciduous teeth – as may occur in cleidocranial dysostosis where the permanent teeth remain unerupted.

(c) Normally it is an isolated anomaly. However, it has been associated with congenital cardiac defects and Down's syndrome.

66 (a) Painful ulcers and erosions.

(b) Treatment for the generalised disease process and local steroid – antibiotic therapy is often helpful.

67 (a) Failure of the right upper central incisor to erupt.

(b) A supernumary tooth in or about the midline of the premaxilla.

(c) Removal of the supernumary tooth is usually rapidly followed by eruption of the delayed incisor.

68 (a) Such patients often develop non-erosive lip lesions – the histology is of lichen planus.

) None.
) Erosions of the lip (usually the lower) which are susceptible to trauma and
ten present a crusted non-specific appearance. Steroid creams are helpful.

 (a) Midline glossitis in one of its variants.
) It is associated with candidal infection.
) Topical antifungal agents – these will improve (without always eliminating) the
sion.

 (a) Enamel hypoplasia.
) At one to two years, approximately.
) It is a marker of coeliac disease, resulting from the disturbance of calcium
etabolism after weaning.
) The strong genetic element involved in coeliac disease warrants a jejeunal
opsy and haematological screening to detect malabsorption.

 (a) Acute leukaemia.
) Primary herpetic stomatitis.
) A full blood count and film survey.
) Abnormal white cells present in viral infections may be mistaken for leukaemic
lls.

 (a) A midline fissure of the lip – not necessarily associated with any other
ndition.
) Staphylococci or candida.
) Local antibiotic treatment may be sufficient. Excision and suture may be
eded eventually as these are often difficult to treat.

3 (a) An evident carcinoma of the floor of the mouth.
) Biopsy with immediate arrangements for definitive treatment.
) Older male patients are much more often affected (ratio 4:1) than similarly
ged females.

4 (a) Leukoplakia of the gingivae and alveolar ridge.
) Relatively minor trauma in a susceptible patient and possibly a genetic element
volved.
) Biopsy to confirm a non-aggressive histology or if a more active process is
own, excision should be carried out.

5 (a) Herpetiform ulceration.
) Multiple small painful ulcers which may coalesce.
) It is often responsive to local tetracyclines but not to steroids.
) As it is often associated with haematological abnormality or flat jejeunal
ucosa, a full haematology screen is needed, followed by jejeunal biopsy if
dicated.

6 (a) Lichen planus.
) Geographic tongue.
) The buccal mucosa may be affected.

7 (a) Acute lymphoblastic leukaemia.
) Gingival enlargement, ulceration and echymosis are the most common.
) Platelet deficiency.

8, 79 (a) An elongated styloid process.
) A granuloma which is palpable from the mouth resulting from pressure of the
yloid process on the soft tissues distal to the pterygoid hamulus.
) Radiating upwards from the soft palate on the side involved.
) Fracture and removal of the inferior part of the elongated styloid.

80 (a) An aspirin burn caused by placing an aspirin tablet in the buccal mucosa next to the tooth causing pain.

(b) The origin of the pain is determined by simple examination – in this case the heavily filled molar.

(c) Treat the cause of pain – the mucosa will rapidly return to normal and antiseptic mouthwashes will eliminate secondary infective factors.

81 (a) Papillary hyperplasia of the palate.

(b) It is unknown although, in this patient pipe and cigarette smoking was excessive. Candidal infection may be present.

(c) Opinions on this vary – from considering it to be a potentially malignant lesion to a relatively innocuous condition. The more conservative approach to this condition is now favoured.

82 (a) Attrition, erosion and abrasion.

(b) An obsessive personality with dietary abnormalities (such as excessive fruit consumption) and exaggerated use of hard toothbrushes.

83 (a) Pyostomatitis gangrenosum.

(b) Pyoderma gangrenosum.

(c) Vasculitis and subsequent tissue necrosis.

(d) Pyostomatitis vegitans – the oral equivalent of pyoderma vegitans (See **153**).

(e) A diffuse stomatitis which may be quite non-specific or may resemble recurrent aphthous ulceration.

84 (a) A papilloma of the palate; palatal polyp, leaf fibroma.

(b) The distortion of structure caused by compression from the denture makes assessment of the tissue of origin difficult. The term 'fibroma' (implying connective tissue neoplasm) is inappropriate.

(c) Simple excision.

85 (a) A full haematological screen including serum iron, folate and B12 estimations.

(b) Deficiencies in folate and B12 as well as latent anaemias. This patient was shown to have pernicious anaemia.

86, 87 (a) Cleido-cranial dysostosis.

(b) Deficient calcification or absence of the clavicles, bossing of the frontal bone and multiple unerupted teeth.

(c) The unerupted teeth may be quite unsuspected – the clinical presentation may be of partial anodontia or of retained deciduous teeth. Extraction of standing teeth may be very difficult because of the unerupted teeth.

(d) A single gene transmitted condition – in many families several members have this condition.

88 (a) The failure of cartilagenous bone to calcify. Enamel and dentine may show abnormalities.

(b) Vitamin D.

(c) 20-30 per cent have enamel hypoplasia, as this patient.

(d) Osteomalacia – this may be a primary deficiency disease or secondary to other diseases (or therapy) which affect calcium metabolism.

89 (a) Gemination of the left lower lateral incisor.

(b) Deciduous dentition.

(c) The incisors and occasionally the premolars.

90 (a) No, this ampicillin rash is not necessarily associated with general penicillin hypersensitivity.

(b) Glandular fever (infective mononucleosis), although this is unsubstantiated.

91 (a) Macrocytosis, anisocytosis and poiklocytosis.

(b) Serum vitamin B12 estimations, tests for the presence of parietal cell antibodies and folate levels. If abnormalities are found, a Schilling test to determine B12 absorption function.

(c) Pernicious anaemia, although folate deficiency may result in a similar blood film.

92 (a) Gingival hyperostosis – a condition ranging from minimal local gingival bone enlargement to the widespread condition shown.

(b) None – it is an isolated developmental phenomenon. Paget's disease could be an alternative diagnosis if the condition had just presented, but this rarely occurs in patients younger than 40 years.

(c) None.

93 (a) Partial anodontia (hypodontia).

(b) Ectodermal syndromes – anhydriotic ectodermal dysplasia being the most common. However, then the teeth frequently show abnormal morphology – often being peg shaped.

(c) No.

(d) Lower second premolars, upper lateral incisors and upper second premolars (in that order).

94 (a) Denture granuloma (denture induced hyperplasia).

(b) Epithelialised scar tissue.

(c) It is thought to be an entirely benign lesion.

95 (a) Although, evidently, a number of possible differential diagnoses including various forms of neoplasia should be considered, this is most likely to be a simple fibro – epithelial polyp.

(b) These lesions are most often seen on the buccal and lingual mucosa but the dorsum of the tongue is not a rare site.

(c) As in all lesions of this kind, simple and conservative excision.

96 (a) Geographic tongue.

(b) Unusual, but not rare.

(c) In younger patients there is often considerable distress – usually in relation to eating or drinking.

(d) None.

97 (a) Echymosis of the palate.

(b) Platelet deficiency.

(c) Acute leukaemia.

(d) Often, patients with a common cold or sore throat may present with a very similar appearance.

98 (a) Acute ulcerative gingivitis.

(b) Gingival soreness, bleeding, general malaise and halitosis.

(c) Unknown.

(d) *Borrelia vincenti* and *fusiformis fusiformis* are invariably present although it has never been shown that these are causative.

(e) Any debilitating disease may predispose, although most patients have no such background.

99 (a) Computerised axial tomography (CAT) in both coronal and sagittal planes in the head.

(b) In neoplastic and other space filling and displacing lesions.

(c) It is a space filling parotid lesion (in this case a lymphoma).

100 (a) Attrition.

(b) There is occlusal dysharmony which is associated with temporo-mandibular pain dysfunction problems.

(c) No, although it is a well known cause of temporo-mandibular joint dysfunction.

101 (a) Squamous cell carcinoma.
(b) In the early stages the prognosis is good, but in a lesion of this size the involvement of lymph nodes becomes much more likely and therapy more difficult.
(c) 20:1.
(d) 20:1 in males, less in females.

102 (a) Cyclic neutropenia.
(b) The cyclic nature of the neutropenia should be confirmed by serial blood screening.
(c) Neutrophil production defects.
(d) Drug induction.

103 (a) Median glossitis – a more proliferative form than in **69**.
(b) Carcinoma of the tongue although this presentation is not typical.
(c) If doubt remains, yes. In this case the clinical appearance does not suggest malignancy.
(d) Antifungal treatment as it is usually associated with candidal infection.

104 (a) Scleroderma – the lips may become hard and immobile.
(b) Widening of the periodontal ligament.
(c) Female.

105 (a) Retained deciduous second maxillary incisors.
(b) Absence of the permanent successors (hypodontia).
(c) Yes. The maxillary second incisors are the most frequently absent permanent teeth after the lower second premolars.

106 (a) A retention cyst of the submandibular duct is the most likely diagnosis.
(b) A calculus impacted at the duct orifice.
(c) Simple radiography to confirm calculus formation. However, non calcified 'calculi' may also cause obstruction.
(d) If a calculus cannot be extruded, then incision of the swelling and retrograde removal of the calculus is necessary.

107 (a) A 'pipe smokers palate' – tobacco smoking induced lesion.
(b) Pipe smoking rather than any other tobacco habit.
(c) Good, with no evidence of malignant transformation, although persistent benign ulceration caused by breakdown of an inflamed palatal mucous gland may be troublesome.
(d) Leukoplakia in other sites, particularly the floor of the mouth.

108 (a) The buccal lesions of Crohn's disease.
(b) Biopsy.
(c) Non-caseating tuberculoid granulomas in the lesions.
(d) For gastrointestinal tract abnormalities and for malabsorption (see **12**).
(e) Yes, most patients with oral Crohn's disease present at about this age.

109 (a) Expansion of the right maxillary sinus.
(b) Facial contour is more readily seen than in a frontal view.
(c) From above the head downwards – the reverse of this view.
(d) Carcinoma of the antrum.

110 (a) Herpes simplex lesions.
(b) In a herpetic patient the giving of a nerve block anaesthetic or the trauma of dental treatment may precipitate such lesions.
(c) No treatment is likely to affect the course of the lesions at this stage.

111 (a) Gingival fibromatosis with hypertrichosis.
(b) Mental retardation or epilepsy.
(c) It is transmitted as an autosomal dominant disorder.

12 (a) A torus palatinus – a simple abnormality of bone growth.
b) None – it is an entirely local phenomenon.
c) None, unless problems arise in providing a denture.
d) A pleomorphic adenoma.

13 (a) Gingival pemphigoid.
b) Biopsy with immunofluorescent studies – in pemphigoid deposits of IgG, IgA or C3 may be found in a linear distribution at or about the basal zone.
c) The eyes should be examined for the presence of early lesions.

14 (a) Typical lesions of lichen planus.
b) Skin and oral lesions may occur separately or together. They may be separated by a considerable period of time.
c) Any site on the skin, but frequently on the flexor surfaces of the wrists.
d) Nine months is an average for skin lesions – oral lesions are often present for years.

15 (a) Blue sclera – the result of choroid pigment showing through a deficient sclera.
b) Osteogenesis imperfecta.
c) There are two major forms. In the less severe form there is autosomal dominant transmission with a variable degree of penetrance. The other form has a recessive mode of transmission, resulting in multiple fractures and deformities.
d) Dentinogenisis imperfecta of both primary and secondary dentitions.

16 (a) The so-called 'brown hairy tongue' resulting from gross elongation of the filiform papillae.
b) In some cases it follows a course of antibiotic therapy.
c) There is no fully satisfactory treatment available but most cases spontaneously regress after a variable interval.
d) It is unknown.

17 (a) Perioral eczema.
b) Local steroids – to prevent atrophic changes in the facial skin 1 per cent hydrocortisone cream is usually recommended.
c) Eczema and angular cheilitis of Crohn's disease are the only lesions of this kind which respond to steroids. In other forms of angular cheilitis steroids are contra-indicated.

18 (a) The onset of a squamous cell carcinoma in a pre-existing area of lichen planus.
b) No.
c) Erosive lichen planus – in this case, the carcinoma arose in a non-eroded area.

19 (a) These ulcers are usually larger than the minor variety, and they persist for several weeks or months, healing with scarring and frequently affecting the oro-pharynx.
b) Aphthous ulcers in the floor of the mouth or in the depths of the buccal sulcus often present in this elongated form.
c) Oro-genital ulceration or, with other systems involved, in Behçet's syndrome.
d) No fully effective treatment. Relatively high doses of systemic steroids usually suppress the ulcers but with side effects. High concentration local steroid therapy may avoid this problem.

20 (a) Acute pseudomembranous candidiasis (thrush) superimposed on the healing erythema multiforme.
b) Candidiasis may occur during treatment with either local steroids or local antibiotics. The combination of the two makes this more likely.
c) Local antifungal treatment.
d) Antifungals may be used as a prophylactic measure.

121 (a) Herpangina.
(b) Usually (but not invariably) children.
(c) Only a minor degree of systemic upset but in a few patients fever and malaise, sometimes with abdominal pain, are more severe although transient.
(d) A viral parotitis resembling mumps.
(e) Hand-foot-mouth disease, although it is more commonly associated with the Coxsakie A16 type virus (see **27, 28**).

122 (a) Conical teeth may be associated with hypodontia of any degree. These teeth may represent a half-way stage to total suppression.
(b) Ectodermal dysplasias but may also occur without this association.
(c) The maxillary lateral incisor. A conically shaped lateral on one side is often associated with its absence opposite.

123 (a) Fordyce's spots – normal sebaceous glands in the oral mucosa.
(b) When the mouth is sore and erythematous (for instance, during the course of common cold) the glands stand out in contrast to the rest of the mucosa. Under these circumstances it is also more likely the mouth will be self-examined and the structures noticed.
(c) Confusion with abnormal structures.

124 (a) Denture stomatitis.
(b) A chronic atrophic candidiasis affecting the palate below a denture.
(c) 'Denture sore mouth' – although the condition is painless.
(d) None. It is an entirely local condition.

125 (a) A traumatic keratosis.
(b) No, it is not considered premalignant.
(c) Nothing other than long term observation.

126, 127 (a) The typical appearance of a pipe smoker's palate – a diffuse white palatal mucosa with distended mucous glands.
(b) No – in European smoking habits it is not considered premalignant. In cultures with differing habits, the prognosis is less good.
(c) Acute pseudomembranous candidiasis – thrush.
(d) Oral candidiasis often occurs in incompletely controlled diabetes, so the degree of stability of the diabetes should be assessed, starting with a random plasma glucose estimation. Well controlled diabetic patients are also susceptible to candidiasis, here the combination of tissue trauma from smoking and susceptibility to candida infections produced the condition.

128, 129 (a) Pemphigus and pemphigoid are the most likely – dermatitis herpetiformis is a possibility.
(b) Biopsy with immunofluorescent studies is the most important diagnostic manoeuvre.
(c) Although pemphigoid (in all its variants) and dermatitis herpetiformis may cause problems, pemphigus is a fatal disease unless treated promptly and aggressively.
(d) Over 60 per cent of patients with pemphigus develop oral bullae before skin lesions. Early treatment greatly reduces the effect of the eventual skin lesions.

130 (a) A papilloma.
(b) The tongue, followed by the palate. Viral warts (which are clinically indistinguishable) occur often on the lips following inoculation from warts on the fingers.
(c) Papillomas occur at any age; more frequently in females.

131 (a) Diffuse melanosis of the buccal mucosa.
(b) Endocrine abnormalities – in particular Addison's disease (hypoadrenocorticism).
(c) Candidiasis.

(d) It may occur as a reaction to a wide range of drugs including antimalarials, hormones (such as oral contraceptives) and cytostatic drugs.
(e) Melanin is often deposited in the corium below the lesions of oral lichen planus and may persist after the primary lesions have resolved. Other disturbances of oral epithelial structure may invoke the same response.

132 (a) 'Midline rhomboid glossitis' (see **69**).
(b) This was considered a remnant of the embryonic 'tuberculum impar' – the site where an ingrowth of epithelium occurs to eventually form the thyroid gland.
(c) Chronic candidal infection.
(d) Local antifungal treatment helps.

133 (a) Denture stomatitis associated wtih a full upper denture with a palatal relief chamber.
(b) Two – trauma from long term wearing the denture and candidal infection. Systemic disease is rarely involved.
(c) None – the alternative term 'denture sore mouth', is a misnomer.
(d) Angular cheilitis.
(e) Prosthetic – the provision of satisfactory dentures, perhaps with the use of tissue conditioners as an initial step. Antifungal treatment to the palate may be helpful and careful cleaning of the dentures, which often carry a surface reservoir of candida, is essential.

134 (a) The so called puberty gingivitis.
(b) This represents an enhancement of the response of the gingivae to the presence of plaque as a result of the endocrine changes during puberty.
(c) It occurs more frequently and earlier in girls.
(d) Strict oral hygiene measures are the basis.

135 (a) 'Idiopathic oral blood blisters', originally known as 'angina bullosa haemorrhagica'. It is presumed that there is some weakness of the basal zone of the oral epithelium resulting in the formation of blood-filled blisters but the mechanism involved is obscure.
(b) Mucosal pemphigoid is the most obvious. In pemphigoid the blisters are filled with clear fluid – but occasionally this may become blood-stained from secondary haemorrhage.
(c) Biopsy with immunoflorescent studies. In this condition no diagnostic immunological findings have been described. The immunological findings in pemphigoid are strongly indicative, but not entirely diagnostic since in some cases immune complexes cannot be demonstrated at the basal zone.
(d) No preventive treatment is available. Large bullae may be incised, often by the patients themselves.

136 (a) Hyperkeratosis of the soles (tylosis). The palms are usually also involved.
(b) Keratosis of the attached gingivae.
(c) In the Papillon-Lefevre syndrome it is associated with rapid periodontal destruction in childhood leading to early loss of both the deciduous and permanent dentitions.
(d) Occasionally it is associated with oral leukoplakia and a marked tendency to develop oesophageal carcinoma (see **52, 53**).
(e) It is transmitted as an autosomal recessive characteristic.

137 (a) An enlarged pituitary fossa.
(b) Protrusion of the mandible.
(c) A pituitary adenoma leading to acromegaly.
(d) Prognathism, coarsening of the face and enlarged hands and feet. These may all occur before any primary signs or symptoms of the pituitary lesion become evident. Secondary symptoms of temporomandibular joint disturbance arising from excessive mandibular growth, were the earliest indication of the problem.

138, 139 (a) Neoplasia must be considered when otherwise unexplained proliferative or ulcerative lesions occur in the mouth. The history and appearance of **138** strongly suggests neoplasia while **139** implies an infective origin.

(b) Identification by biopsy followed by definitive surgery. There is no evidence that biopsy of minor salivary gland neoplasms may be followed by malignant change. In **138**, when biopsy showed an adenocystic carcinoma, there would be no other way to plan the extent of surgery.

(c) The lesion (**139**) is a palatal sinus resulting from the drainage of an acute periapical abscess on the first maxillary molar. Firstly, identify and extract the tooth – with antibiotic cover if necessary. Rarely would further action be needed.

140 (a) An advanced stage of 'pipe smokers palate' (see **107**) in which palatal mucous glands have broken down to produce ulcerative lesions.

(b) In terms of potential malignancy it remains good, but the ulcers may be very persistent.

(c) Discontinuing the smoking habit will help, but it takes time before the mucosa returns to normal. A covering plate may be helpful but may cause trauma unless very carefully constructed.

141 (a) A diffuse lymphangioma.

(b) It is a benign naevus involving the lymph vessels and behaves in an essentially static manner in most cases.

(c) Yes.

(d) Yes, most cases are diagnosed before twenty years of age.

142 (a) Atrophic candidiasis.

(b) Melanosis associated with the Addison's disease (see **131**).

(c) It is one manifestation of the endocrine-candidiasis association and the result of the abnormal immune response. Pseudomembranous candidiasis or mucoco-cutaneous candidiasis may occur.

(d) These are three manifestations of autoimmune processes which occasionally present together.

143 (a) A mucous cyst (mucocele).

(b) Either extravasation of mucous from a mucous gland into the surrounding tissue or obstruction of a mucous gland duct.

(c) Trauma.

(d) A haemangioma (because of the rather blue colour and the dilated capillaries in the cyst wall).

144 (a) Crohn's disease – oedema, fissures and granulomatous tags may occur in both sites (see **12**).

(b) Examination of the gastrointestinal tract by contrast radiography, even in the absence of symptoms of gut disease.

(c) Minimal complaints of irritation.

(d) Both respond readily to local steroids.

145 (a) 'Pregnancy gingivitis' with an associated 'pregnancy epulis'.

(b) An exaggerated response to plaque resulting from enhanced progesterone levels.

(c) The 'pregnancy epulis' is very likely to have the histological appearance of an immature granuloma with many primitive blood vessels.

(d) As it is likely to resolve to a great extent after pregnancy and it is not causing interference with occlusion or other problems, it is best left. After the pregnancy excise the remaining lesion which now consists of more mature tissue and will be relatively simple to handle.

(e) Strict oral hygiene measures.

(f) Resolution after pregnancy if strict oral hygiene measures are maintained.

146, 147 (a) Wegener's granulomatosis.

(b) In the early stages a characteristic granulomatous gingivitis may occur.

(c) Predominantly younger male patients (M:F=2:1).

(d) Vigorous steroid and immunosuppressive therapy may save the patient in what was previously a fatal disease.

148 (a) The result of the proliferation of a wide range of bacterial organisms – often not otherwise considered to be pathogens (compare with **48**).

(b) Isolation of the responsible organism and sensitivity determination.

(c) The appropriate antibiotic must be used systemically and locally. Disintegration of the bacterial plaque by trypsinisation helps to clear the infection.

149 (a) Minor aphthous ulceration – although this diagnosis would depend as much upon the history as on the appearance of a single ulcer.

(b) Malabsorption, increased demand (as in pregnancy) or dietary factors. Some forms of drug therapy (particularly phenytoin) and a high alcohol intake may also lead to lowered folate levels.

(c) The serum folate level indicates the current status of the patient – it is a labile measurement which can vary from day to day and be changed by a single meal. The red cell folate level is an indication of the folate included in the red cells at formation. This remains unchanged during the life of the erythrocytes and is thus a more stable measure, giving an indication of long-term folate status.

(d) In a very few patients aphthous ulceration is a direct consequence of folate deficiency and may be eliminated by folic acid treatment.

(e) In 6 per cent of patients the jejunal mucosa is found to be flat as in coeliac disease (see **61, 62**). Many of these patients have lowered folate levels as a marker of malabsorption.

(f) Jejunal biopsy.

(g) If the jejunal mucosa is flat, a gluten free diet will eliminate the oral ulceration. Other forms of malabsorption should be considered before folic acid supplements are given.

150 (a) Paget's disease.

(b) Blood chemistry determinations which would show a considerably increased alkaline phosphatase level. Urinary hydroxyproline levels would be raised. Further, more specialised, biochemical investigation should follow.

(c) There are two types of facial pain. Compression of the foramina of the skull may cause a neuralgia like pain with a recognisable anatomical distribution. A more diffuse 'bone pain', not limited to the distribution of any nerve, may also occur.

151 (a) It has the typical distribution and haemorrhagic appearance of herpes zoster affecting the second division of the trigeminal nerve.

(b) Post herpetic neuralgia which may be distressing and intractable to treatment.

(c) Immediate treatment with anti-viral agents – 40 per cent Idoxuridine in Dimethylsulphoxide or Acyclovir for the skin lesions.

(d) Blood dyscrasias – in particular leukaemias and agranulocytosis.

152 (a) Anatomical – their extent and distribution varies widely.

(b) None, however, they may be noticed by the patient on self-examination and considered important.

(c) Superficial infections may begin in the region of fissures – presumably as a result of the relative stasis in their depths. Conditions which may result in a generally sore tongue (such as anaemias) may present initially with soreness along the fissures. Non-painful lesions (such as hairy tongue) also apparently may begin and spread from sites adjoining fissures.

(d) In long-standing inflammatory conditions affecting the tongue – particularly in chronic candidiasis – the morphology of the tongue may become grossly distorted with the formation of non-anatomical fissures. The clinical picture is quite different from the situation shown here (see **18**).

119

(e) There is very mild angular cheilitis present – in the absence of any evident reason for this a haematology screen would be indicated. If the tongue were to become sore the need for this would be evident.

153 (a) Pyostomatitis vegetans – the result of the coalescence of intra-epithelial micro-abscesses. The mechanism of formation is not known although, histologically there is an eosinophilic perivascular infiltration in the dermis.
(b) On the skin – pyoderma vegetans.
(c) Pyostomatitis gangrenosum may occur in some patients with ulcerative colitis (see **83**).

154 (a) Homogenous leukoplakia – in the terms of the accepted WHO definition which implies a lesion which is not susceptible to any other clinical diagnosis.
(b) Biopsy and assessment of the degree of epithelial atypia.
(c) Excision and grafting or laser excision dependent upon the biopsy result. Cryotherapy is somewhat less satisfactory in the treatment of homogenous leukoplakia than in speckled leukoplakia.

155 (a) 'Desquamative gingivitis'.
(b) The inflammatory changes present in most 'normal' gingival tissue make the interpretation of gingival biopsies difficult.
(c) Pemphigoid.
(d) Lichen planus (see **58**). Both gingival lichen planus and gingival pemphigoid may produce this clinical picture without other mucosal involvement, although diagnostic histological or immunological changes may be found in the nearby mucosa.

156 (a) Erythroplakia is of greatest significance.
(b) Treatment depends entirely upon the results of a representative biopsy.
(c) If significant epithelial atypia are shown in the biopsy material then adequate surgical removal should be considered. If not, close observation is the minimum action.
(d) The red areas of erythroplakia, histologically associated with increased epithelial atypia in many cases, are said to be the frequent site of malignant transformation.

157 (a) Exfoliative cheilitis.
(b) Earlier descriptions suggested it was part of the atopic picture but there is no known real association with other disease processes.
(c) None, however, it seems to be a self-limiting condition.

158, 159 (a) Erythema multiforme
(b) Intact bullae are present (see **60** for a typical presentation).
(c) Local steroids and antibiotics.
(d) Recurrent episodes are likely. The interval is unpredictable and variable However, if herpes is a precipitating factor an attack of erythema multiforme may be expected to follow a facial lesion of herpes.
(e) Idoxuridine or other antiviral agents may abort or diminish the severity of the episode.

160 (a) Connective tissue disease – here, mixed connective tissue disease, a condition with a variable range of signs and symptoms which might be present in lupus erythematosis, polymyositis or scleroderma.
(b) Biopsy. The histology was not of lichen planus, as might have been expected, but was similar to that in connective tissue diseases (see **25**).
(c) A full immunological investigation. The distribution of antinuclear antibodies varies characteristically (but not absolutely diagnostically) in this group of diseases. Anti-ribonucleoprotein antibody is indicative of mixed connective tissue disease.
(d) Systemic steroid therapy.

161 (a) A diffuse haemangioma of the tongue.
(b) Mixed haemangioma-lymphangiomas. This does not affect their management.
(c) None, unless there are problems of haemorrhage or soreness. Surgery is difficult but cryosurgery is often more effective.

162, 163 (a) Sjögren's syndrome associated with SLE as the connective tissue disease component rather than the more usual rheumatoid arthritis (see **50, 55**).
(b) Antinuclear antibodies, LE factor and anti-RNA and DNA antibodies. Only 50 per cent of patients with Sjögren's syndrome have anti-salivary gland antibodies.
(c) Most patients developing SLE are female and between the ages of 10 and 40 years.
(d) Only moisturising mouthwashes or similar preparations are useful in relieving the oral dryness. In the eyes, obtunding the lachrimal drainage may be very helpful.

164 (a) A clinical diagnosis is almost impossible – a number of neoplastic or inflammatory lesions may occasionally appear in this site. This is a simple fibro-epithelial polyp in an unusual situation (compare with **95**).
(b) Squamous cell carcinoma. This site is a very unusual one for carcinoma – in contrast to other parts of the tongue.
(c) Diagnosis depends on biopsy – biopsy excision might be the best procedure.

165 (a) Epistaxis (bleeding from the nose).
(b) The nasal mucosa – particulary that of the nasal septum – is often involved in erythema multiforme. Frank epistaxis is uncommon – erythema and erosion of the mucosa is more usual.
(c) Bullous diseases which affect the oral mucosa – particularly pemphigoid and pemphius.

166, 167 (a) Dystrophic epidermolysis bullosa.
(b) Extreme fragility of the skin resulting from disturbance of the sub-epithelial tissue structure. Loss of epidermal appendages follows.
(c) Mucosal instability paralleling that of the skin and, often, some degree of enamel hypoplaia. Oral hygiene, therefore, is difficult to attain.
(d) The susceptibility to caries, the difficulty in maintaining oral hygiene because of the fragile mucosa, the difficulty of applying anaesthetic techniques (again, because of skin and mucosal fragility) and the restriction in mouth opening because of scarring.

168 (a) A fibroepithelial polyp.
(b) Lipomas or salivary adenenomas may have a similar appearance.
(c) Very local excision biopsy. The histological examination will indicate if more active surgery may be considered.
(d) The term 'fibroma' implies a true connective tissue neoplasm while these lesions are almost certainly an inflammatory reaction to chronic trauma.

169 (a) Another variant of geographic tongue (see **30, 64**).
(b) Chocolate and cheese are two of the most commonly mentioned irritants in this condition, although the reason is unknown.
(c) Very little – reassurance is most important.

170 (a) Melanotic spots on the buccal mucosa.
(b) Endocrine abnormalities are the most likely systemic association (see **131**).
(c) 'Oral melanotic macules' is a term suggested for such idiopathic melanin production.
(d) None. The number of melanocytes is normal – the production of melanin is increased in the affected areas for some unknown reason.

171 (a) A cheek chewing habit.
(b) There is no long-term adverse effect in most cases. In some patients with psychiatric abnormalities the degree of self-mutilation may become gross.
(c) A simple covering appliance over the teeth may help to break the habit.

172, 173 (a) Oral candidiasis – in this case part of an endocrine-candidiasis syndrome. In **172** pseudomembranous candidiasis of the palate (thrush) is present.

(b) A deficient immune system which shows a particularly poor response to candidal infections. Muco-cutaneous candidiasis may result – but, in this case, oral candidiasis only.

(c) Treatment of Addison's disease with corticosteroids is replacement therapy – the immune deficiency is not improved by this.

(d) An early candida leukoplakia.

(e) Long-term treatment with antifungals (at the present time Imidazoles are the most successful) will help to reduce the candidal infection, although permanent elimination is unlikely. The potential for malignant transformation of candidal leukoplakias should be kept in mind.

174 (a) Squamous cell carcinoma of the buccal mucosa.

(b) Approximately 15 per cent of all oral carcinomas involve the buccal mucosa.

(c) Leukoplakia is said to precede carcinoma in this site.

(d) There is a possibility of regional lymph node involvement with a subsequent lowering of the chances of a long-term successful result, in a lesion of this size.

175 (a) A simple mucous cyst (mucocele).

(b) The site (see **143** for a more common presentation).

176, 177 (a) Post radiation rampant caries.

(b) Lack of oral hygiene (the result of soreness of the mucosa and hypersensitivity of the teeth) and reduced salivary secretion.

(c) As careful oral hygiene measures as possible should be instituted, reinforced by fluoride applications or mouthwashes.

(d) Fibrosis following radiation mucositis.

(e) In this patient few. In an edentulous patient prosthetic problems may be considerable. Traumatic ulceration caused by ill-fitting dentures may involve the underlying relatively avascular bone and osteomyelitis may result. If the masticatory apparatus is involved in the area of fibrosis, trismus may become a considerable problem.

178 (a) Tuberculoid granulomas lying below the epithelium, closely resemble tuberculosis of the skin (lupus vulgaris).

(b) Tubercle organisms must be demonstrated. The demonstration of acid fast organisms by conventional staining techniques is not very satisfactory in the case of oral lesions. Specific fluorescent stains are more useful, but guinea-pig inoculation should be used if doubt remains.

(c) Elimination of systemic disease (in particular pulmonary). Family screening should be conducted.

(d) Long-term anti-tubercular drug therapy, as for pulmonary tuberculosis.

179 (a) The Melkersson-Rosenthal syndrome – aetiology unknown.

(b) A deeply fissured tongue is found in a high proportion of patients.

(c) Non-caseating tuberculoid granulomas similar to those in sarcoid or Crohn's disease.

(d) This is an autosomal dominant transmitted condition.

(e) Oral Crohn's disease is the first alternative diagnosis. It has been suggested that Crohn's disease, sarcoid and this syndrome represent differing facets of a spectrum of disease.

180 (a) Actinomycosis must be considered in view of the induration around the sinus, although there are several possibilities.

(b) The organisms, assuming actinomycosis, should be isolated and sensitivity, with minimum inhibitory concentrations values, determined.

(c) Long-term oral antibiotic treatment is satisfactory if the therapeutic levels are attained.

81 (a) Allergic oedema or hereditary angio-oedema.
(b) If a true allergic reaction cannot be demonstrated then the blood levels of C1 esterase inhibitor and C4 should be assessed. These (particularly C1 esterase inhibitor) are deficient in hereditary angio-oedema.
(c) Prophylactic treatment of hereditary angio-oedema is not generally available, though in some very specialised centres, C1 esterase inhibitor from pooled plasma is available as replacement therapy during severe episodes. Long-term treatment with anabolic steroids has been reported as successful. Tranexamic acid has been used to treat acute episodes. Allergic oedema may be treated by adrenalin (in the acute situation) and by steroids and antihistamines.

82 (a) Chronic candidiasis affecting the nail bed.
(b) Chronic mucocutaneous candidiasis in a relatively restricted form, often affects only the oral mucosa and the finger nails. Other conditions with widespread immune abnormalities, may appear similarly.
(c) Recent systemic antifungals are often effective in clearing the oral candidiasis. The nail deformity response depends on the degree of previous damage.
(d) A wide range. However, deficient T cell function (not number) is the most commonly reported finding.

83 (a) Focal epithelial hyperplasia.
(b) Hyperplasic changes in the epithelium, often with considerable cellular regularities.
(c) Unknown – but there is considerable evidence for a viral aetiology.
(d) Crohn's disease (see **108**).
(e) Most patients (but not all) are children. South African coloureds, Eskimos, American Indians and some Europeans, are among the several racial groups in which this condition has been described.
(f) None is known.
(g) It is self-limiting and eventually spontaneously regresses.

84 (a) Crohn's disease affecting the gingivae.
(b) Biopsy shows non-caseating tuberculoid granulomas as in Crohn's disease in other sites (see **108**).
(c) No local treatment is entirely successful. However, it rarely causes trouble other than mild and transient soreness. Maintenance of oral hygiene standards is very important.

85 (a) Sarcoid.
(b) No, very uncommon.
(c) Antigenic material is prepared from the spleen of a known sarcoid patient and injected intradermally. A characteristic tuberculoid granuloma develops over some six weeks in a positive patient and is identified by skin biopsy.
(d) No specific treatment is normally needed for skin or oral lesions. If the generalised condition warrants it, systemic steroids may be used.
(e) Good in most cases without active pulmonary involvement. In this case the lesions went into spontaneous remission.

86 (a) A leukoplakia – an intrinsic white lesion of the oral mucosa. It has been described in a number of patients on high levels of immunosuppressive treatment.
(b) No reports of malignant transformation has yet been made but in view of the increased incidence of malignancy in general in these patients, they must be considered as potentially dangerous. In this case the lesion regressed with reduction of the drug therapy.
(c) Biopsy to determine the degree of atypia followed by close observation. Here, the histological appearance was reassuring.

187 (a) A spreading herpes simplex infection.

(b) Immune incompetence arising from abnormal lymphocyte function.

(c) In compromised patients with spreading lesions of herpes, vigorous treatmen with currently available local and systemic antiviral agents is justified.

188 (a) Local trauma – when new dentures are provided after a long interval suc effects are common.

(b) A full haematological screen to eliminate the possibility of a systemic backgroun Instability of the lingual mucosa resulting from haematological abnormalities ma help to produce apparently simple traumatic lesions.

(c) If abnormalities show on the haematological screen the treatment must includ correction. If not, the treatment is essentially prosthetic, which may be ver difficult in patients with persistent tongue habits.

189, 190 (a) Viral warts.

(b) Transmission of the papilloma papovavirus from the fingers to the mouth b chewing the finger lesions.

(c) None, mostly. These are self-limiting lesions which regress in 6-12 month Cryotherapy may accelerate the process.

191 (a) Probably Bell's palsy – idiopathic loss of function of the seventh crani nerve. It is a lower motor neurone disturbance.

(b) Determination of whether this is an upper or lower motor neurone abnormalit In the latter case all branches of the facial nerve are affected and there is weakne of the muscles of the forehead which does not occur in upper motor neuron disease.

(c) Pain and tenderness of the parotid region on the affected side.

(d) Early cases may benefit it by short term, high dosage, rapidly reducing system steroid treatment.

192 (a) Preleukoplakia.

(b) This clinical term does not imply any specific histological pattern or any defini prognosis.

(c) Where genetic factors are involved, observation on a long-term basis wit biopsy and surgical intervention if and when indicated. In other circumstance where extrinsic factors (such as a tobacco habit) may be involved, reduction of th stimulus is an evident step to take.

193 (a) The occurrence of rampant caries in occasional diabetic patients is we known. Although it does not usually occur in a reasonably controlled diabetic there are changes in salivary gland function which may explain the increased carie rate.

(b) Strict oral hygiene measures and the reduction of plaque.

(c) Enhanced levels of gingivitis and oral infections (particularly candidiasis, se **53**).

194 (a) Papilloma, verrucous carcinoma or squamous carcinoma should be initiall considered as well as an unusually proliferative simpler keratotic lesion. Biopsy wi determine diagnosis.

(b) The appearance of a proliferative white lesion surrounded by an area o leukoplakia is characteristic of verrucous carcinoma.

(c) Most patients with verrucous carcinoma have a long history of tobacco usage.

(d) This is dependent upon the biopsy result. In the case of verrucous carcinoma local surgical excision followed by careful follow-up, is indicated.

195 (a) Herpes simplex infections only rarely appear with this localised palatal distribution of discrete vesicles.
(b) Coxsackie virus infections are much more likely to present in this way.
(c) None. Approximately 10 per cent of oral herpetic infections are caused by herpes 2 virus. It is not possible to distinguish between the two on clinical grounds.

196 (a) Squamous cell carcinoma.
(b) Biopsy (the diagnosis is not certain on clinical grounds alone) followed by immediate definitive treatment.
(c) Not good as approximately 50 per cent of carcinomas of the lateral margin of the tongue are accompanied by cervical nodes at first presentation.
(d) Most carcinoma of the tongue is in patients over 60 years of age. Recent surveys show an equal sex distribution.

197 (a) Atrophic candidiasis and hairy tongue resulting from the therapy (see **116**, **120**).
(b) If it is essential to continue the steroid-antibiotic regime, an antifungal agent should be added. This will not clear the hairy tongue component which may well resolve on cessation of therapy.
(c) Antifungal therapy in any future regime of this kind.

198 (a) Not at all. It was thought that racial or geographical factors were involved in the distribution of periodontal disease but it is now known that this is not so.
(b) There is a clear relationship in all communities and races between the levels of oral hygiene and the incidence of periodontal disease. Rarely do factors such as nutritional levels play a part.

199 (a) This is a not very marked geographic tongue. The condition has been described as having a high incidence in patients with psoriasis, although the evidence is unconvincing.
(b) A wide variety has been described but the association is very doubtful.
(c) In psoriatic arthropathy the temporo-mandibular joints may be involved resulting in symptoms much like those of rheumatoid arthritis affecting these joints.

200 (a) Ecchymosis as the result of platelet deficiency.
(b) The development of auto-antibodies to platelets.
(c) Ulceration and generalised stomatitis (see **66**).
(d) Most patients are female, and under 20 years of age at the first appearance of symptoms.

Index